THE
FOOD
Therapist

THE
FOOD
Therapist

**BREAK BAD HABITS,
EAT WITH INTENTION,
AND INDULGE WITHOUT
WORRY**

SHIRA LENCHEWSKI, MS, RD

sphere

SPHERE

First published in the US in 2018 by Grand Central Life & Style, an imprint of
Grand Central Publishing, a subsidiary of Hachette Book Group, Inc.

First published in Great Britain in 2018 by Sphere

1 3 5 7 9 10 8 6 4 2

A CIP catalogue record for this book
is available from the British Library.

On page 46, the future self continuity scale © Hal E. Hershfield.

Cover design by Claire Brown
Cover copyright © 2018 by Hachette Book Group, Inc.

ISBN 978-0-7515-7336-7

Printed and bound in Great Britain by
Clays Ltd, St Ives plc

Papers used by Sphere are from well-managed forests
and other responsible sources.

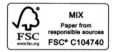

Sphere
An imprint of
Little, Brown Book Group
Carmelite House
50 Victoria Embankment
London EC4Y 0DZ

An Hachette UK Company
www.hachette.co.uk

www.littlebrown.co.uk

For Andrew, of course

Contents

Introduction

If you asked people to post a status update on their relationship with food, I'm guessing most would toggle to "It's complicated." Much like thorny love connections, our relationship with food is one of life's most emotionally loaded, yet still instantly gratifying, bonds. When things are good, they're oh so good—there's passion and excitement, comfort and confidence—the stuff you wouldn't trade for anything. On the other hand, when your interactions feel stagnant or strained, everything seems like a struggle. You may go through periods of second-guessing your every move or maybe even giving up effort entirely. Yet, while any genuine romantic relationship is bound to be somewhat complicated, given that there are built-in issues of trust and fairness along with a second helping of life's problems (since there are two of you), the same doesn't have to be true of your relationship with food.

The interesting thing, though, is that many of us analyze our romantic relationships at length (and—*ahem*—sometimes to death) but don't really spend much time digging deep when it comes to our ongoing relationship with food. But here's the simple truth: You can't make better, more consciously driven food decisions that are in line with what you really want for yourself and ultimately reach your health and bod goals if you don't examine the roots of this vital relationship. And yet, in my experience, most people haven't even skimmed the surface of their personal backstory with food (aside from throwing endless shade at themselves).

When people used to ask me about my interest in nutrition, I'd often tell them about growing up as an athlete (rowing) and my focus on food in terms of fueling my body. While both those things are valid, I realized later that I was leaving out what was in many ways much more important and relevant: the full picture. I was an uber-anxious, self-conscious kid who grew up in the 90s, when the fat-free craze and other gag-worthy diets were alive and well. I grew up hearing about weight a lot—family members saying things like, *Ugh, I'm so fat*, *Look how skinny she is*, etc. I was actually a healthy-looking kid, but I didn't feel good in my own skin. I didn't love my bod, but I did love food, and I thought that you kind of had to pick a lane—you could either feel good about your bod but relinquish the joys of eating delicious food, *or* you could enjoy food but in turn sacrifice having the body you wanted. I genuinely thought it was an either/or thing. Without all the facts, the self-awareness, or the self-compassion, I became the queen of Diet Coke and sad salads with dressing on the side. As I eventually discovered, not only is this a really gloomy way to live, but restricting yourself this way doesn't actually work. It keeps you forever hungry and constantly thinking about food, and quite frankly, I had more important sh*t to do.

Ditching this narrow mindset was a complete and utter game changer, but I couldn't have switched gears without forgiving myself for doing it wrong all those years, for doing the eating equivalent of biking uphill with my brakes on (something I've unfortunately done, by the way). The moral of the story for me was that you don't have to choose between looking and feeling your best *and* eating delicious, flavorful, satisfying food. In fact, I honestly think you've got to have both factors at play to make consciously healthy food choices on the regular. It's the same reason you'll never find me fasting on Yom Kippur (Jewish New Year), doing a liquid cleanse, or engaging in anything ultrarestrictive when it comes to food because, honestly, I've been there and done that, and not only did it feel like crap but it also didn't bring the results I craved. So rest assured: The reason I can speak so definitively about food-related missteps is that I've known them intimately, both personally *and* professionally.

Some details on the professional part: I'm a registered dietitian in private practice in Los Angeles, and I'm more or less a food therapist. Truth be told, the gig wasn't exactly what I was expecting, coming out of my clinical-nutrition graduate program, but I've fully embraced the role. In grad school at NYU, I pored over biochem and organic chemistry with serious gusto. (Not joking; I freaking love science.) But after finishing my dietetic residency at Mount Sinai Hospital in New York City, I realized just how much the science stuff takes a backseat to the emotional aspects in everyday life. In my practice, I work with different types of women and girls (and some dope dudes, too), from editors, law-firm partners, MBA students, middle-schoolers, high-schoolers, and Hollywood folk to working moms and full-time moms—a varied and unique bunch, to say the least. Early on, I noticed a recurring theme that's still ongoing today: Most of my clients can immediately rattle off all the things they *ought* to be doing: limiting added sugar, exercising portion control, making better choices at restaurants, etc. The problem is that they're not actually doing those things on a regular basis. In other words, there's a gap between their intentions to get healthier or lose weight and their day-to-day eating behaviors. So before my clients and I get to the actual meal planning, the crux of our initial work plays out more like a food therapy session, getting to the bottom of *why* they aren't doing those things.

But how is it that so many of us are motivated to look and feel better *and* understand the basics needed to get there, and yet we're not following through? Hint: It's *not* because we're the worst (although, ironically, that's often where our heads go). It's largely because the vast majority of us have a conflict-ridden relationship with food. When you add up the emotional baggage that comes with that troubled-relationship territory, the constant distractions we all deal with on the daily, and the physiological issues involved, it's not actually all that shocking that we're not delivering on our get-healthy goals. The reality is, it's really difficult to translate our good intentions into effective actions in the face of all this noise, because we're constantly working against ourselves.

Here's the awesome news: It's scientifically proven that at any age, we can change the way our brains function to boost willpower and develop consistent healthy habits and behaviors, *even* if those habits and behaviors don't necessarily come naturally to us. But we can only get there if we're willing to flex different mental muscles and practice these moves on a regular basis. The first step in developing healthy behaviors is to identify your personal roadblocks and then to phase out your emotional hang-ups around food and your body. After that, you can start applying strategies to help you deal with these root causes in order to make truly thoughtful eating choices that serve your ultimate goals, whatever they may be.

And *that* is exactly what you're going to learn to do in this book. Part One is like a one-on-one food therapy session, where I'll help you broaden your understanding of your personal history with food, what makes you tick (and eat), when you tend to lose control, and what your values are in terms of indulgence and pleasure. You'll begin by pinpointing the factors that cause you to stray from your healthy-eating intentions so you can use that info as a road map to anticipate and sidestep those obstacles in the future. Then you'll learn how to develop workable food-related coping strategies that will better serve you—including how to tune in to your body's signals (no ashram required) and employ willpower more efficiently so it's available when you really need it. In Part Two, I'll map out the Food Therapist Plan for getting your hormones working for you, including meal plans, recipes, and strategies for keeping this plan sustainable and enjoyable for the long haul. I'll also help you develop tools that will enable you to bounce back quickly when things go amiss (this is real life, after all). All of this will help you set yourself up to execute new behaviors that will become habits—and keep honoring them long after the New Year or that beach vacation.

By the time you've finished this book, you will have gained a permanent spot in the driver's seat. Rather than allowing your emotions, your environment, or other factors to dictate what or how much you eat, you'll be in charge of your own food decisions. I'm also certain that you, too, have way better things to do than stress about food. *It's on.*

PART ONE

YOUR DIG-DEEP FOOD THERAPY SESSION

1

Time to Have *The Talk* with Yourself

Hit the pause button on your regularly scheduled life for a few moments and let's get right into it. Let me ask you something: How do you talk to yourself when it comes to food and your body? Better question: Would you let anyone else speak to you that way? What about when you happen to overdo it on sweets or comfort foods, or anything, for that matter? Do you tend to think of your eating habits as *good* or *bad, virtuous* or *naughty*? Better question: Do you think of *yourself* in those absolute terms based on what or how much you eat?

Like most complicated relationships, our connection with food is seriously layered, and it's tied to what is arguably the *most* complex bond of all: the one we have with ourselves. Anyone who has been in a grown-ass romantic relationship knows that the more intimately you know someone, the more clearly you see his or her flaws. It's easy to love someone when things are ultrasmooth. Ride-or-die love is different: It's *choosing* to love and be committed to the person, *despite* his or her faults. That can be scary (and challenging). I'm not talking about quirky faux flaws that aren't really deficits (like being a neat freak or a bed hog); I'm talking about the messier stuff, like the way your loved one acts when he or she is under enormous pressure or feeling particularly down. Depending on you and your significant other, seeing that ungraceful, possibly disappointing, twisty stuff can be a total deal-breaker.

With respect to our relationship with *ourselves*, we don't really have that luxury. We can't simply peace out (*it's not you, it's me*–style) when we overeat or aren't thrilled with our bods. Instead, we tend to put ourselves in the dog-house when we'd be so much better off approaching those disappointments compassionately, just like we do when our favorite people let us down. In my mind, ride-or-die love in a healthy, sustainable relationship means two imperfect people refusing to give up on each other. It's a pretty amazing thing we do, not only for romantic partners, but also for our BFFs and other people we care about and believe in. So why is it that we rarely afford ourselves the same tolerance and TLC, *especially* when it comes to eating and our bodies? Ideally, we should all be striving for that kind of bond and ability to accept imperfections with ourselves, too—not only because it feels better, but also because it's part of the secret sauce that helps us close the intention-action gap between wanting to eat healthier and making consciously healthy choices on the daily. So imagine taking a vow to make that same commitment to *yourself*: on bloated days *and* skinny-jean days; after a particularly indulgent month and post–sugar cleanse, too. This doesn't mean you have to love your bad habits or even your cellulite for that matter, but you do need to accept that they are a part of you and your story (at least for now). It sounds touchy-feely, I know, but stay with me. Ironically, once you accept yourself this way, without the shame and negativity that fogs up your perspective mirror, *then* you can figure out your roadblocks and start working on stuff that's actually in your power to improve. As a starting point, it's wise to examine how well you tune in to and treat yourself on a day-to-day basis—how well you listen to your wants, figure out your needs, and dish out self-compassion, all of which affect the quality of your relationship with yourself.

You're probably thinking, this all sounds fine, but what does it have to do with food? Well, that care (or lack thereof) also influences your relationship with food, playing a central role in what, why, and how much you eat, and how you feel about it. The fact is, the foods we choose and the way we eat are very much tied to the way we think about our bodies (for instance, *My stomach is gross* or *I hate my thighs*) and the way we speak to ourselves (*I have no self-control* or *I'm such a sloth*), especially when we stray from our good intentions. Same thing goes for the way we understand our food histories (including ghosts of diets past). Having a healthy relationship with food means being on our own team—for real, though, not just when we're at our fittest and most together.

What I've found, again and again, in working with my clients is that approaching food relationships this way, and accepting our food-related fumbles without the typical shame spiral, allows us to identify and really get to work on overcoming the obstacles holding us back from making solid food choices consistently, day in and day out. This is major, because before you can change your food behavior, you've got to be willing to confront why you're not already practicing the healthy habits you want. Over the years, in my private nutrition-counseling practice, I've seen clusters of patterns that reflect why clients weren't applying the food behaviors they aimed to carry out, as well as how and when they were veering off course. The most common obstacles include having trust issues related to food, being a pleaser (as in: caving to other people's food choices in order to keep the peace), having a *go-big-or-go-home* mindset when it comes to dining, craving a bit too much control around food, being hot and cold with noshing habits, and using food as a vehicle to amplify good feelings and temporarily forget about bad ones. When I work with clients, we always start out by exploring their specific eating obstacles and tendencies. And that's exactly what we're going to do here—only, in this case, you'll do a self-compassionate deep dive on yourself.

It's time, then, to DTR (define the relationship). Anyone who has ever teetered in the uncomfy are-we-exclusive gray area while dating can agree that it's best to approach *the talk* as straightforwardly as humanly possible, because quite frankly, it's important to know where you stand. The same is true of your relationship with food. As psychologist Kelly McGonigal puts it in *The Willpower Instinct*, "The best way to improve self-control is to understand how and why you lose control." That's what I'm talking about here: In order to change your eating behavior, you'll need to zoom in on where you are now and explore how you got here. As with any relationship, it can be difficult to confront your emotional baggage and missteps along the way, but remember: The goal isn't to punish yourself for these missteps, but to understand how, when, and why you've ditched your long-term goals for your more immediate wants; this is the crucial first step to closing the gap between your intentions and actions. To set the wheels of change in motion, I developed the following DTR quiz that will help you investigate the underpinnings of your relationship with food and what's been holding you back.

Once you complete this quiz, there's a good chance you'll identify with a couple of different obstacle types. That's normal—it's part of what makes you unique. The aim of exploring the patterns found in each of those obstacle categories is to spark some introspection about why you've been making the food choices you have. In doing so, you can start recognizing patterns that don't work for you or that may be standing in your way of making healthy changes that last. It's almost like once you start thinking about your "problematic tendencies" without the accompanying scary music, dealing with your eating-related baggage doesn't feel so intimidating, and you can focus your energy on gathering strategies to help you deal. (I want to make something crystal clear, though: I am not talking about eating disorders here; I'm talking about the everyday issues we all have with food.)

Without further ado, let's dive in.

QUIZ: WHAT ARE YOUR FOOD-RELATED HANG-UPS?

To suss out the food-related obstacles you struggle with most often, read the following statements under each category and check the ones that describe you.

TRUST ISSUES

____ Family-style dinners and buffets are beyond tough for me; I often lose restraint and end up overeating, big time.

____ I try not to keep sweets or starchy snacks or _____ [fill in the blank] at home, because I'm afraid I'll eat them all. In fact, I know I will.

_____ I'm not personally familiar with willpower; somehow, I just didn't get that gene.

_____ I know the basics of healthy eating, but I don't trust myself to make good decisions with food.

_____ I don't feel in tune with my body; I'm not always sure when I'm hungry or when I've had enough—I just don't know my limits.

_____ Despite my good intentions, I frequently find myself eating foods I shouldn't or simply too much. It's a problem.

THE PLEASER TRAP

_____ When eating with other people, I tend to go with the flow and let my dining companions take the lead in choosing (and ordering) food.

_____ I prefer not to ruffle feathers in general, so when it comes to dining out I don't like to be a burden and ask questions about the menu or request modifications.

_____ Making other people feel comfortable is very important to me, and I've been known to put other people's wants and needs before my own.

_____ You could say I'm a bit of a chameleon when it comes to my eating habits; I like to fit in and tend to mirror my dining companions' habits.

_____ When friends or family members want me to eat more or sample something I'm just not into, I often feel at their mercy and cave in.

(continued on next page)

_____ I like to make people happy and would never want someone to be bummed out by my food choices. Basically, I don't want to let anyone down.

FEAR OF THE MUNDANE

_____ For me, dining out (and eating, in general) provides an opportunity to really let loose and enjoy myself. I feel like I'm selling myself short if I don't indulge to the absolute fullest.

_____ Quite frankly, eating healthfully or limiting myself sounds like a huge bummer. Eating delicious food is one of the greatest joys in my life.

_____ I like what my go-big-or-go-home eating style represents—my fun-loving, adventurous, spontaneous side—and I think other people appreciate that about me, too. It's one of my signature qualities.

_____ I'm a thrill-seeker, and I can't stand the idea of food monotony.

_____ I work hard, so I want to play hard, too, and that means eating whatever I want to.

_____ Sometimes I worry that if I revamped my eating habits, people would think of me as less fun or likable.

A CRAVING FOR CONTROL

_____ Generally, I am a rule-follower; as far as I'm concerned, the more rules the better when it comes to food and other lifestyle decisions.

____ Eating the same things every day makes me feel like all is right in the world. My routine gives me a sense of order.

____ There are some foods I just won't let myself eat because left to my own devices, I'm worried I would completely lose it.

____ I don't expect to love everything I eat, and that's cool with me. Consistency is key.

____ I get mad at myself when I overindulge or eat the wrong things. I'm intimately familiar with food guilt.

____ Being *good* is important to me, and sticking to my food rules makes me feel like I'm honoring that.

A HOT-AND-COLD PATTERN

____ I'm not a halfway kind of person: I'm either totally obsessed with what I'm doing or completely disinterested.

____ I often get really amped about starting a new project but struggle with maintaining interest after the newness fades.

____ I have a history of serial dieting; I love trying out the latest health trends and food fads but rarely stick with them.

____ Generally, I feel motivated to eat healthfully, but ultimately my environment drives what I eat; I often go with what's convenient or with foods that seduce me with their irresistible aromas and good looks.

(continued on next page)

_____ Sometimes I jump into projects without fully thinking them through or understanding why a particular approach or undertaking makes sense for me.

_____ I often tell myself what I should or shouldn't be doing based on what other people are doing.

A DEPENDENCE ISSUE

_____ I tend to use delicious indulgences as a way to treat myself—to make myself feel better when I'm bummed out or to celebrate victories.

_____ I often find myself snacking when I'm procrastinating.

_____ When I'm really down or emotionally frayed, I often have trouble controlling my eating; I tend to continue noshing to soothe myself even after I'm full.

_____ When it comes to food, I tend to live in the here and now and eat what's going to make me feel good in the moment.

_____ I hate feeling emotionally out of sorts; having good food often cheers me up and makes me feel better in ways that few other things can.

_____ I often use food to help me cope with upsetting situations or unsettling feelings; this can help temporarily, but it often leads to overeating and then I end up feeling even more upset later on.

If you chose two or more from any of these obstacle patterns, read all the corresponding analyses that apply to you, below. This will give you some insights into why you've been struggling with the food issues you have. Hey, there's no judgment here! We all have issues—and our own unique combos of them—so the challenge is to understand them, find tools to cope, and learn to live with them in a healthy way that doesn't suck to maintain. It's possible, *I promise.*

TRUST ISSUES

You don't always trust yourself around food. Maybe you don't keep certain foods like sweets or chips at home because you're afraid you'll eat them all. Or maybe you dread family-style meals because you usually leave them feeling stuffed beyond reason. Like many of us, you probably learned to associate food with comfort and rewards as a kid—thanks to ice cream cones after a bad day and pizza for celebrations—and now it's your go-to for both. At the root of these issues is the fact that you may not trust your inner system of checks and balances; in other words, you may be out of touch with your body's hunger and satiety signals.

You may even be what I call a *perma-dieter*: individuals who have a history of trying lots of different diets, many of which were restrictive and unsustainable. The cycle goes something like this: they followed the strict guidelines initially, making some weight-loss progress, but eventually fell off the plan *hard*, reversing the progress they made. At that point, feeling terrible about themselves but determined to do better, they began the cycle again with another unsustainable diet. And so on and so forth, reinforcing the ultimate disservice: mistrust in their own food judgment and self-control. In fact, research shows that many perpetual dieters are somewhat desensitized to their internal fullness signals; as a result, their food behavior is often driven by external or environmental forces. This may sound like a stormy forecast for the future, but it really doesn't have to be (for real).

THE PLEASER TRAP

Like a mirror, you tend to reflect the behaviors of the people around you (in general, but especially with food). When it comes to food, this means you often let other people drive your choices. You may think you're being agreeable or go-with-the-flow but if we're being honest, you're also habitually relinquishing control of what you put in your body. You're definitely not alone. A pair of studies published in the *Journal of Social and Clinical Psychology* found that people with a strong desire to please others and maintain social harmony eat more when they believe their dining companion wants them to.

The trouble is, you're the third wheel in your relationship with food. Having this profile makes it endlessly challenging to stand up to inadvertent sabotage and food pushers who, for whatever reason, want you to eat more or indulge in certain things. Plus, when you constantly cater to what other people want you to eat, it's hard to know what *you* actually want and need. This may add to your own stress and frustration. It's time to realize that putting yourself first in this way doesn't make you high maintenance. You'll need to challenge this notion in order to get the results you crave.

FEAR OF THE MUNDANE

You're somewhat of a maximalist, with a go-big-or-go-home mindset. You probably work hard, deal with a lot of pressure (at work, home, or somewhere else), and food is one of the main ways you treat yourself—by ordering the most decadent thing on the menu or by indulging in foods that may not be healthy but give you a major pleasure rush. With some of my clients, this mentality is a huge part of how they move through the world and connect with other people. So the idea of having to reel in your carefree and adventurous culinary spirit may feel like an assault to your identity. I get that—really, I do. You may even be worried that if people start seeing you eating more healthfully, you'll get unwanted attention for *that*—and worse, if you don't stick with it, everyone will know.

The truth is, you may be overly invested in food as a source of pleasure and reward, whether it's because you're not getting pleasure in other ways or your high stress load makes you crave not just the taste of decadent food, but also the temporary soothing effect it can have. Behavioral scientists acknowledge that a major stimulus for noshing isn't actually hunger, but the anticipated pleasure of enjoying highly palatable foods. This may be especially true for you, and even more so during stressful times. After all, increased cortisol exposure from chronic stress can amp up the brain's reward system, making the drive for these super-palatable foods even stronger. The problem isn't that you love delicious food—that's actually *fantastic*—it's that your food choices are primarily driven by this reward-seeking behavior, which can hijack your ability to think big-picture.

A CRAVING FOR CONTROL

Your hyper-disciplined eating habits may make you feel like you're on top of your game, but between your lists of good foods and forbidden ones and your tendency to be especially hard on yourself, you're probably not enjoying your meals all that much—and that's a major bummer, to say the least. To keep yourself on track, you might eat the same things day after day, meal after meal. You stick with what you know and feel comfortable with, but this Groundhog Day technique not only comes at the expense of really taking pleasure in the food you're eating, it also gives you a false sense of calm, when it actually causes more stress (and undue stress at that). Not to mention, it's counterproductive. Without realizing it, exercising strong cognitive dietary restraint (when you obsess over what or how much you should or shouldn't eat) can amp up your stress hormones (hello, cortisol), causing you to crave sugar and overeat. As it happens, a 1994 study published in *Appetite* found that rigid eaters are actually *more* likely to lose control around food than their more flexible counterparts.

Whether this pattern stems from anxiety, stress overload, or a previous history of feeling out of control with food, one thing's for sure: It's destined to make you feel like complete and utter crap. The trouble is, you don't know how to deal with food any other way. Complicating matters, if you've adhered to restrictive diets in the past, your body's internal regulatory cues (the ones that tell you when you're physiologically hungry and when you've had enough) may be seriously out of whack. It makes sense if you think about it, because in order to follow a drastic diet you've practiced telling your brain not to listen to your body, and over time the brain follows suit.

A HOT-AND-COLD PATTERN

When it comes to dating, you don't always crave the same thing. Sometimes there's nothing better than having the comfort of a steady love interest; other times, you lust for the excitement of playing the field. This conundrum can also happen with food: Sometimes you're motivated to eat healthfully; other days...not so much. While you may like the idea of losing weight or giving your diet a wholesome makeover, you may not have fully committed to making it happen. More often than not, your environment tends to drive what you eat, meaning that despite having legitimate healthy-eating goals, you often go with what's convenient or what looks good in the moment. Oftentimes these behaviors are so ingrained and automatic that it's nearly impossible to make real changes unless you're willing to welcome some serious self-awareness. Maybe you're ambivalent about the undertaking. Or perhaps you don't have clarity about what you really want or why you want it, so you may have major conflicting desires at play. Either way, it's important to figure out what's truly motivating you and why you want to make these changes for the long haul. It may be that you're primarily motivated by extrinsic reasons (because someone told you that you should, for example) instead of intrinsic ones that are personally important to you (because *you* want to look and feel your best). Intrinsic reasons transcend external ones any day of the week.

It's time to do a little soul-searching. Think about what you really want and what's standing in your way of totally going for it. Sometimes wanting to get healthy is a notion that gets thrown around, almost like offering to help someone move: It sounds good in theory, and it may be something you think you *should* want to do (or that a partner, friend, or parent wants you to do). Also consider: Are you afraid you'll fail if you jump in with both feet? Or perhaps, and sometimes even scarier, are you afraid that you'll succeed and then you'll be forced to deal with the other stuff in your self-improvement queue? Once you figure out where you stand on these issues, you'll be in a better position to weigh your long-term goals against your right-now desires and improve your eating habits consistently.

A DEPENDENCE ISSUE

Food serves as a crutch for a whole lot of feelings for you: good, bad, and everything in between. Maybe you were taught to use food as a reward as a kid (getting a lollipop after a shot at the doctor's office) or a way to self-soothe (after a fight with a friend), and you've applied that pattern to grown-up issues, too. Consciously or not, you've come to associate certain food-related rewards with being the most efficient route to feeling good. It could be that when your stress meter is in overdrive, you feel especially out of control with food, because you may not have many other coping strategies to turn to. Or you may unconsciously try to blunt or soften feelings of discomfort or distress by eating because it's always done the trick. One way or another, food has become your go-to remedy. This, my friend, is extremely common, but it's not in your best interest.

It's true that food provides short-term relief from unpleasant feelings, physically and emotionally. For one thing, eating may distract you from what's bothering you; for another, consuming delicious (particularly sweet and starchy) foods can light up the pleasure center of your brain like a pinball machine, offering a serotonin boost that dulls bad feelings in the moment. But eating for emotional reasons just doesn't work long term because you often end up overeating, and then feeling even more stressed about *that*. Anyone who identifies here is probably familiar with this overeat-repent-repeat effect, but you may not realize how it plays out big-picture. Several studies suggest that when people try to alleviate distress by eating, they can also check out emotionally, which leads to less self-awareness and more disinhibited eating over time. Not really the plan, right?

TAMING THESE TENDENCIES

Let me make something 100 percent clear: There's no need to sweat it if any of this is striking a painful chord. The truth is, everyone struggles with this stuff: It's human nature because roadblocks aren't personal failures—they are an inherent part of the human condition. In his book *F*ck Feelings*, psychiatrist Michael Bennett puts it perfectly, stating, "There's always something that can, at least temporarily, overwhelm human control and cause us to do things we'll regret, and believing otherwise only makes us more foolishly vulnerable." This is true when it comes to eating as much as anything else, so let's stop punishing ourselves for having weaknesses and instead learn how to live with them. Many of us believe that if we were "good" or "strong" enough that we could have complete control over temptations and food cravings, but that's just not real life. But when we understand the nature of our limits and stumbling blocks, then we can figure out how to manage them, and that's the goal here.

Now that you have a better idea of what the underlying issues are in your connection with food, you can take steps to address them in specific and effective ways. If you just discovered that you struggle with multiple obstacles, don't panic; oftentimes these patterns have plenty in common. For example, trust issues, a craving for control, dependence issues, and a hot-and-cold pattern are often driven by a lack of confidence in your own food judgment and exacerbated by negative self-talk; in contrast, a fear of the mundane, a hot-and-cold pattern, dependence issues, and a craving for control tend to be driven by intense or unprocessed emotions. Meanwhile, the pleaser trap, a fear of the mundane, and a craving for control can be influenced by individual personality factors and values, while the pleaser trap, trust issues, a fear of the mundane, and a hot-and-cold pattern are often driven by your response to other people and environmental cues.

Sometimes an illustration is worth a gazillion words. So for you infographic lovers, here's a Venn diagram to illuminate the big picture. If the thought of Venn diagrams takes you back to middle school in a bad way, don't stress. The main point here is to show the natural relationships and overlapping qualities between these different obstacle patterns:

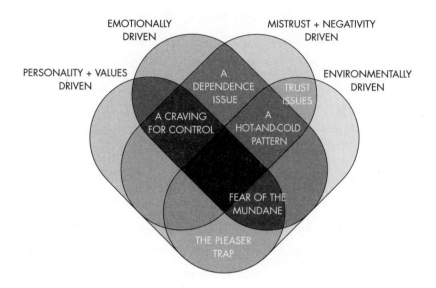

It seems complicated, I know. But the point is, most of our major healthy-eating roadblocks are at least in part overlapping and interconnected because we're all susceptible to a wide range of influences that can throw us off course. These forces lead us to overeat and employ not-so-great hand-to-mouth behaviors that prioritize our right-now desires over our long-term goals, keeping us stuck in neutral (or reverse). The reality is that these forces will always be there, so it's up to you to get better at anticipating them and identifying your personal vulnerabilities in order to start making conscious eating choices that are in sync with your ultimate goals. *That* is precisely what you're going to gain from the coming chapters. In Chapter 2, you'll learn how to take additional steps to unpack your emotional food baggage so you can use those insights to propel yourself forward.

2

Cutting to the Core of Your Emotional Hang-ups Around Food

We all have vulnerabilities and insecurities, memories and associations that play out in myriad ways when it comes to our love lives *and* our eating habits, and I'm pretty sure that's an inevitable part of being human. It's rare to meet someone who thinks about food purely in terms of its most basic function—as a source of life-sustaining nourishment and pleasure. For most of us, food and eating in general are infinitely charged subjects. Think about it: Beyond using food as a way to nurture and bond with the people we love, it's also a pretty powerful symbol of security and comfort, reward and good times, and even courtship and seduction (*oysters, anyone?*).

Like most things in life, our food-related behaviors have

personal and cultural roots. We adopt them by observing the people who raise us and share our homes, by watching friends and peers, and by seeing food and eating norms play out in the media. Over time, we learn that eating is one way to assert our unique tastes and preferences (i.e., the great cilantro divide: People either love it or hate it), and in that respect, individual food choices can be used as a way to express who we are and what our deal is. We're also shaped by the beliefs and attitudes we hear on the regular: that certain foods and eating behaviors have the ability to make us *more* or *less* attractive; that some foods are "good" and others are "bad"; and that people with self-control around food are virtuous winners and those without are impulsive plebs. Even the term "table manners" implies there's a *right* and a *wrong* way to eat (and doing it wrong is at *best* impolite). As 19th-century scholar D'Arcy Wentworth Thompson famously wrote in his book *On Growth and Form*, "Everything is the way it is because it got that way"—which sounds kind of cryptic, but really just means that we observe, interpret, and learn from these patterns, put our own spin on them, and eventually they become our own.

Time to ditch the Anthro 101 lecture and get to the point: For most of us, what we choose to eat (and *not* eat) is a loaded decision, whether we realize it or not. When you hear about tragic breakups, there are, of course, stories of betrayal and drama, but oftentimes they involve a slow and quiet demise of the relationship: one small misunderstanding after another.

Distance develops. In the end, there's enough distance that it can't be ignored. Not to be a downer, but that's kind of how I see emotional food issues playing out. Time after time, we feel low-key disappointment in ourselves but fail to examine the root causes, and ultimately we just lose faith in our ability to make healthy changes and achieve our goals. So we don't. *This doesn't mean we're all screwed.* But these emotional hang-ups can certainly throw us off course when it comes to eating healthfully consistently, so the key is to prevent obstacles and detours from stopping us in our tracks.

ENDING THE BLAME GAME

The trouble is, many of us respond to personal eating setbacks by waging war on ourselves—with relentless criticism, followed by some combo of guilt, shame, and apathy. Anyone who has experienced this particularly uncomfy emotional blend knows it's *seriously* stressful. Not only does this draconian tactic feel terrible, it also does not work. When we try to scold ourselves into shape, it often backfires, sapping our motivation to pick up and try again. In those vulnerable moments, we're not thinking about how to learn from our missteps; we're too busy trying to feel less annoyed, so we often head straight to our feel-good foods for temporary relief. This phenomenon is real enough to warrant a legit formal, scientific name—counter-regulatory eating—but researchers also refer to it as the *what-the-hell effect*: When people view a (minor) detour from their dietary intentions—such as having a piece of pizza or a cupcake—as a colossal failure, the synergy of guilt, shame, and frustration they experience leads to a false sense of helplessness. Then, they end up throwing caution to the wind and eat whatever the hell they want. This set-up can lead to a cycle of indulgence they then regret, followed by even greater indulgence and more regret, and so on. Instead of finishing a slice of pizza and closing the box for the night, a shame-ridden person might say, "What the hell, I already ruined everything. I might as well polish off the whole pie."

Any perceived setback can send this negative cascade into motion. In a study published in a 1998 issue of the *Journal of Abnormal Psychology*, researchers at the University of Toronto rigged a scale to make restrained eaters and non-restrained eaters believe they were five pounds heavier or lighter than they actually were. As you may have guessed, restrained eaters who were told they were carrying an extra five pounds felt depressed, guilty, and utterly disappointed in themselves. Non-restrained eaters weren't as vulnerable to these emotional effects. And not all that surprisingly, when the restrained eaters were presented with a subsequent "taste test," they ate significantly more food than the other groups did—an example of the *what-the-hell effect* in action.

Take my former client Jason, an ad exec, as an example: He's a total food maven, with a serious appreciation for the finer (read: *fancier*) things in life. Yet, he couldn't stop eating his kids' stale Halloween candy one December. He would do it in private and hide the wrappers from his wife and kids out of utter shame. In our sessions, we delved deeper, and I mentioned that based on his history of loving the finer things, this pattern didn't totally add up—after all, he wasn't eating artisanal chocolates, but instead vintage Tootsie Rolls that were hard enough to cleave a tooth. It turned out that he was getting completely buried at work, resulting in stress that triggered cravings for sweets, and at night when he thought about everything he needed to accomplish the next day, he would lose control and inhale leftover candy after his family went to sleep. The kicker: *He wasn't even enjoying it.*

The first step for him was to stop judging himself for wanting a treat and to drop the debilitating shame game. We discussed what it would mean for him to get some high-quality dark chocolate truffles and eat one after lunch or dinner, shame-free, and savor the absolute *$%^&* out of it. When the proposition was presented this way, enjoying something sweet wasn't a naughty act. After eating the truffle, nothing was ruined, and when he took the time to enjoy it slowly and savor the flavor, it was so rich and delicious that he really didn't need a second one (on most days). Having self-compassion and creating a thoughtful game plan for his cravings sidelined the paralyzing guilt and shame and freed him up to really enjoy a treat, then move on.

IT'S PERSONAL

As Jason discovered, if you want to change or improve your eating habits, extracting yourself from the shame spiral is an absolute must. This is challenging because people often take their dietary failures personally, as if they reveal something deeply unsavory and flawed about their character. We also tend to interpret eating setbacks in terms of absolutes, as in "I'm an absolute failure." This black-and-white thinking makes it hard *not* to take dietary indiscretions personally, because they're often perceived as a complete and total loss of control, rather than as a not-so-great yet also not life-alteringly terrible moment in time. In our society, self-control and willpower are viewed as the ultimate virtues, so if you haven't been able to effectively control your food behavior, the faulty yet pervasive myth is that you have no control whatsoever. This leads to poor self-efficacy—the sense that you don't have the will *or* the way to achieve what you want—which can create a self-fulfilling prophecy of not achieving your get-healthy goals. But I assure you: It doesn't have to play out like this.

To put things in perspective, think of it this way: If you had to kick your last partner to the curb because you were being treated poorly, does that make you total garbage at love? *Exactly.* The same is true for failed food relationships from the past. Yet we often take these lapses personally and incorporate them into the way we see ourselves; then we beat ourselves up and end up feeling lousy and destined for loser-dom. On the flip side, if you encourage yourself to view lapses as a result of your *efforts*, rather than character flaws—signs that you're weak and incompetent, for example—you'll be more likely to learn from your not-so-healthy eating behaviors and improve your approach. By contrast, when people attribute healthy-eating setbacks to a lack of *ability* rather than to, say, not planning properly or making the right effort, they're much more likely to quit when the going gets tough.

As any history professor or CEO will tell you, failure has the ability to teach us a lot. In fact, many argue that failure isn't just instructive and normal; it's *vital*. But why is it that while we certainly *can* learn from healthy-eating detours, they often end up making us feel like downtrodden wimps? Well, for starters, how we perceive personal setbacks like these matters big-time. The solution: Cultivating self-compassion can help you clap back at your inner self-critic in ways that will actually improve your eating behavior. I'm serious. As an example, consider this: If you tell yourself "I overate at dinner because I have no self-control," you're much less inclined to improve your approach; in contrast, acknowledging that "I overate at dinner because I didn't really plan properly or I wasn't actually paying attention" gives you something specific and constructive to work on. It's about reframing the reasons you didn't eat the way you planned and focusing on how to improve your strategy in the future.

Contrary to public perception, self-compassion isn't some kind of New Age-y hall pass that encourages free-for-all eating; it actually helps *keep* impulsive eating behavior at bay. Self-compassion is really a matter of treating yourself with kindness, not harsh criticism and side-eye, when things don't go as planned. People assume that being hyper-self-critical keeps us in check, and that if we practice *too* much compassion around food or the state of our bodies, we'll lose our edge and let it all go. But it's actually quite the opposite, because shame and feelings of inadequacy are common triggers for reward-seeking behavior (read: sugar-bingeing) that isn't in sync with our big-picture goals. One major reason self-compassion helps people recover from perceived food fumbles is that without the shame spiral, the *what-the-hell* cycle basically has nowhere to go, because you don't need to escape the unpleasant feelings that typically follow.

In this way, having self-compassion doesn't promote more unconscious indulgences; rather, it makes it easier to approach eating missteps with curiosity, to learn from them, and then do better next time. Sounds pretty good, right? When you disappoint yourself with your eating behavior, instead of throwing shade and raising your voice (inside your head), get *analytical*. The goal is to become aware of what your emotional stumbling blocks are and how they affect your food choices; this way, you can learn from setbacks, rather than letting them kibosh your progress.

In the previous chapter, you zeroed in on your primary obstacles concerning food and how they impact your eating behavior. The next challenge is to figure out how to use those insights to propel yourself forward. For starters, you'll need to rewrite the script that's playing in your head on loop.

Here's how to do it with each obstacle:

TRUST ISSUES

Presumably you have some clue about what lies beneath your trust issues with food, whether it's not having faith in your ability to make good food choices, not being able to rely on your body's hunger and fullness cues, or being easily led astray by external influences. In any case, part of rewriting your story involves dropping the shame and relentless self-criticism, and changing the dialogue inside your head. You might switch from, "I'm a total failure when it comes to self-control" to "Clearly, the eating approaches I've tried in the past haven't worked for me; now I need to figure out why." In the same way that you're not a failure at love because you haven't been successful at maintaining a healthy romantic relationship in the past, people with this obstacle just haven't been in the *right* relationship with food.

Recognizing how the *perma-dieting* cycle (see page 13) has been holding you back should help put things in perspective: It's not that you don't have self-control; it's more likely that you're perpetually distracted and not in tune with your internal hunger and fullness signals, so you're constantly being driven to eat by forces other than legitimate hunger (i.e., big portions, family-style dinner spreads, miscellaneous drama, what's in your cabinets). Part of the fix here is to slow down, get better at listening to your body's internal cues, and keep pre-portioned healthy stuff like roasted nuts and crudités on hand to help you manage between-meal hunger.

THE PLEASER TRAP

No need to get down on yourself, but there's something you should hear: Sacrificing your own get-healthy goals, needs, and desires for someone else's interests may make you feel *nice*—but it can also position you as an emotionally intelligent doormat. Besides, although dining with other people can be an incredible bonding experience, that aspect flies out the window when you completely mirror your companions' eating behavior, because you essentially become invisible. Since you've made a habit of hushing your own desires, you probably have an especially hard time figuring out when you're actually hungry or full and pinpointing what you crave. And since you're so tuned in to your dining companions' vibes and needs, there's a good chance you often feel quite stressed while eating, making it extra difficult to avoid *over*eating.

The reality is, sometimes adopting healthier eating habits *can* shake up social dynamics, but that has absolutely nothing to do with you. It's possible that your partner or your friends may feel like your newfound healthy habits are silently nagging *them* to make changes; or seeing you swing into action may kick up feelings of insecurity if they haven't gotten there yet. But while it's natural to empathize with their struggles, quite frankly, this is on them. As psychologist Edward Abramson has noted, people's body weight can sometimes serve as a sort of equilibrium in relationships, meaning that when one person loses weight and the other does not, it can throw the dynamic off balance and cause conflict. But this isn't your fault, either.

Ultimately, if avoiding this type of conflict is more important to you than achieving *your* get-healthy goals, you're not likely to achieve them. But if you're willing to think about these issues differently, *well*, then you're in business. Forgive yourself for taking a passive role in the past, then let yourself be okay with disappointing people when it comes to dining. If your BFF wants to order dessert and you don't, he or she should go ahead and do that, and if your friend has a prickly reaction, it's probably because he or she is rethinking *their* food choices, *not* because you suck to be around. So forget the notion that prioritizing your needs makes you a pain in the butt. *Cool?* Stick to your guns—and focus on what *you* really want from a meal. When you're dining out, check the menu beforehand when possible and opt to order first so your dining companions won't sway your choices.

FEAR OF THE MUNDANE

People with this obstacle don't usually have to do as much reckoning with the past as they do with the present and the future. Oftentimes I find that those who view decadent dining as the ultimate reward and healthy food as a serious downgrade haven't fully explored how delicious healthy foods—particularly veggies—can be. I'm not talking sad, wilted airport salads, but deliciously seasoned and dressed veggies that will (literally) make your mouth water. If you're willing to expand your flavor-palate horizons, there's a good chance you'll come to see your food choices differently and changing course won't feel like such a bummer. Often it's about challenging notions of what healthy foods are (*not* flaccid steamed veggies or a rubbery, skinless chicken breast).

It's also important to understand that ordering roast chicken with a big green salad instead of a giant plate of pasta doesn't change who you are identity-wise, and choosing a healthier option isn't a punishment. Revising your food history requires being open to challenging your old way of doing things. Instead of telling yourself that you don't like healthy food, you might consider that perhaps you have an outdated idea of what healthy food is, or that you haven't actually had delicious, well-prepared healthy food. Instead of assuming that if you don't eat with abandon you'll be depriving yourself, you might come to view eating healthfully as a reward in itself; after all, you'll be taking good care of yourself, and you're bound to feel pretty freaking great in return. Remember in high school how the very thought of your crush made it easier to get out of bed in the morning? It probably made actual school more enjoyable, too. The key is to channel this drive we all have for wanting to feel good and use it to our advantage by directing it toward behaviors we actually want to make into habits. The easiest way to achieve this is to pair a desired eating behavior with a non-food reward that feels truly awesome. So, if you killed it with portion control on a particular day, or you crushed it with meal prep for the week, reward yourself with something that feels amazing that has absolutely nothing to do with food (such as going for a massage, getting a blowout, taking a long walk with a friend, or downloading a new playlist); this way, you'll start to associate taking good care of yourself with healthy feel-good perks.

A CRAVING FOR CONTROL

Although being critical of your bod and food choices may seem like an effective way to keep yourself in line, it's absolutely crucial that you ease up. Drill-sergeant obedience and monk-like self-denial aren't the goals here; in fact, that type of thinking isn't just unpleasant, it can really trip you up, making it harder to listen to your body's hunger and fullness cues. The truth is, there are no perfect or imperfect days when it comes to food, and thinking this way just sets you up to have a falling out with yourself. As far as get-healthy goals go, there's a huge difference between aiming for perfection and aiming for *your* personal best. The irony of striving for perfection is that it's often what screws up our ability to succeed by skewing our perspective and making us focus on the wrong target; plus, it's an energy drain. Striving for your personal best, on the other hand, leaves room for flexibility and eventual slip-ups with your food choices and eating behaviors. This is essential for every human on planet earth, *even* the most Type A overachievers among us.

Also, consider the beliefs fueling your current approach. Maybe you think you *need* to deprive yourself in order to maintain healthy habits or lose weight, but this "no pain, no gain" mentality is completely unnecessary and prevents you from really enjoying food. Plus, this approach often backfires because the more restrictive we are, the more obsessive we become about food. It's human nature to want (sometimes *desperately*!) what we *can't* have. This is why most people I work with who identify with this obstacle have a history of thinking about food *all the time*. Imagine what you could do with all that extra headspace! If you're willing to loosen the reins of restraint by building in conscious indulgences, you'll be well on your way to achieving what you want—only this time, in a way you can actually sustain.

A HOT-AND-COLD PATTERN

At the root of your on-again-off-again relationship with healthy eating, you may have commitment phobia or some ambivalence about giving your diet a wholesome upgrade. While you may have been lured by certain healthy-eating plans in the past, you probably weren't 100 percent clear on why they were right for you; it could have even been the novelty that appealed to you most of all. Or, like many people, you may have committed to a set of unrealistic goals, and the disappointment of not following through has kept the shame spiral in perpetual motion for you. As a result, it's conceivable you don't believe you have what it takes to make healthy changes.

Now you have an opportunity to change that dynamic by clarifying what you want and why you want it, and then rooting those goals in realistic behaviors. If you're not all that confident in your ability to make healthy changes, why not focus on one specific, small goal, like eating two servings of vegetables a day for three days straight? Following through won't have anything to do with your innate ability to succeed, but instead it *will* depend on the effort you put into figuring out where the veggie servings will fit in and what they'll consist of. So go ahead, and prove your doubts wrong.

A DEPENDENCE ISSUE

So you've developed a habit of leaning on food when times are tough or using it to celebrate when things are going well—you're in good company! Rest assured: It's not a sign of weakness; it's a sign that you don't have the most effective strategies in place to deal with big emotions. The real conundrum with this pattern is that it sets you up to overeat and then feel even more stressed about *that*. Instead of eating because you're experiencing real physiological hunger, a lot of times you end up noshing when underlying emotions or external forces drive you to eat.

As you move forward, try to anticipate potential obstacles that could throw you off course. For example, if you know that having houseguests or attending holiday dinners inevitably leads to overeating for you, prepare yourself with a game plan beforehand. You can also combat these emotional eating cues by introducing ways to treat yourself that have absolutely nothing to do with food (think: massages, foam rolling, infrared saunas, acupuncture, and other forms of bodywork). I'm talking about developing a healthy self-care system, which is a hot topic in the wellness world these days. The self-care umbrella can mean a lot of different things, but basically comes down to prioritizing and doing stuff that makes you feel balanced enough to meet the inevitable stressors of daily living. *And who doesn't need that?*

MIND OVER APPETITE

For better or worse, the way we think about and perceive certain foods affects how we respond to them. In a famous study published in a 2011 issue of *Health Psychology*, researchers from Yale University gave participants different milk shakes on two different occasions: One was described as indulgent and containing 620 calories, while the other was described as sensible and 140 calories. When the participants were led to believe the milk shake was decadent and high-calorie, their levels of the hormone ghrelin (which stimulates hunger) dropped dramatically after they consumed it. By contrast, when they were convinced the milk shake was sensible, their ghrelin levels stayed fairly flat, indicating that they weren't fully satisfied with the lighter, "guilt-free" version. Here's the real shocker: Without knowing it, the participants were given the same 380-calorie milk shake both times.

The takeaway: Our thoughts can legitimately trump our physiology when it comes to food. The participants' hormone levels were influenced by how hungry or full they *thought they should be*; the way they perceived how decadent the milk shakes were affected how satisfied they were by them. This suggests that changing your mindset about certain foods can actually change your body's response to them. *Pretty wild, right?*

RESETTING YOUR MINDSET

In the real world, not the lab, there are quite a few forces working against us when it comes to choosing foods that are in line with our long-term goals, but changing our mindset about healthy foods (and unhealthy ones) can certainly help. If you're constantly fantasizing about sweets and not so interested in veggies, do yourself a favor and stop thinking about sweets as the ultimate indulgence and meals where veggies replace pasta or simple starches as a form of deprivation or punishment. In other words, if you adjust how you *view* healthy foods (in a positive direction), you may be more likely to select and genuinely enjoy them; meanwhile, if you switch up how you think about unhealthy but enticing foods, it may become easier to forgo them. If you're skeptical on the veggie front, be prepared to come around when you hit the recipe section in Chapter 7.

Just as doomed romantic relationships can teach us a lot about what we want, what we need, what's a deal-breaker, and what makes us tick, the same is true of our former relationships with food. So it's time to figure out what went wrong in the past, to identify factors that drive you to make food choices that aren't in line with your big-picture goals, and then forgive yourself. We know it's unhealthy to relive past heartbreaks over and over again, so why do we do exactly that with ex-diets? Let's learn what we can from the past and then leave it behind so we can move on and get to work closing the intention-action gap. Another great perk of letting go of your food-related baggage is that it can help clear the deck so you can focus on other things that really matter to you.

Having a clear sense of what you want and value is obviously a critical step for establishing healthy romantic partnerships in order to make sure you're both on the same page. The same is true of your relationship with food. When you gain clarity about what you want and what you expect from a behavior shift, it's easier to weed out BS goals, things we think we *should* be doing but don't actually plan on carrying out because they reflect other people's values or priorities, not our own. It's kind of like offering to help your casual hookup partner move, even though you have zero intention of getting anywhere near that disaster zone. For example, some people say they *ought* to be cooking dinner from scratch every night or going completely sugar-free, but truthfully this isn't realistic for them and they can't really imagine themselves doing it—these are faux goals with empty promises that should be ditched. In the next chapter, you'll learn how to envision the kind of relationship you want to have with food in the future and how to set yourself up to make that happen—in ways that work for you, on *your* terms, not because you think you *should* be doing it some other way.

3

Meet Your Future Self

When it comes to romantic partners, we lust for someone who's mysterious and spontaneous, but we also want a dependable teammate we can count on when life gives us lemons (*and* to procure feminine hygiene products in a pinch). Similarly, with our food choices, we want to avoid excess added sugar because we'd love to look and feel our best; on the other hand, when we're stressed at work the pull for free office pastries is, well...*palpable*. We pledge to make sensible choices at restaurants in order to achieve our get-healthy goals, but at the same time we want to be able to let loose and really indulge. Oftentimes, the more immediate wants win, and it's *not* because we're all losers. It's because, for many of us, there's a major disconnect between the way we think about ourselves right now and the way we view ourselves in the future. Plus, the human brain is wired to have a strong penchant for sweet and starchy—it's a survival mechanism, *not a design flaw*, because in primitive times it was a serious challenge for our ancestors to find enough to eat. It's just that our modern brains haven't gotten the memo that we now live in a world of excess.

Between our natural drive for palatable sweet and starchy foods and the immediate gratification those foods offer, we tend to be much more focused on making ourselves feel good in the here and now than on anything else. Behavioralists call this a *present bias*, meaning that we often *over*-focus on rewards we can reap right now and neglect to consider ones we might experience in the future. Part of the reason is that, unlike the promise of immediate perks (like the pleasure rush from a donut), down-the-road payoffs don't always feel all that real. It's kind of like texting and driving, which we know is horribly dangerous, and yet so many non-horrible people do it anyway: It's not like people dismiss the potential risks involved because they're laissez-faire about the value of life or wouldn't care about endangering others, but in *that* particular moment they're much more focused on reading or sending a text than on some unfavorable consequence that isn't even certain to happen. On the flip side, I'd bet that same potential injury risk wouldn't be as easy to ignore if they had been rattled by a prior texting-and-driving-related accident. Of course, the stakes aren't nearly as high when it comes to eating, but as you can imagine, our present bias also impacts our food choices. For starters, eating a sweet or starchy treat is *much* more pleasure-inducing in the moment than, say, reading or sending a text message is; plus, the feel-good results from eating healthfully aren't always instantaneous. What's more, when choosing foods, you're less likely to consider the future payoffs from eating healthfully now if you don't actually believe there's a connection between what you eat today and how you'll feel next month. You're also less likely to prioritize your future get-healthy goals if you don't actually think you have what it takes to make consistent choices to help you get there.

Now, let's pivot and focus on the future: A substantial amount of research suggests that the way we think about ourselves in the future can seriously influence our day-to-day food choices. The problem is, many of us feel estranged from our future selves, so we don't make food choices in the moment that are in our best interest for the long haul. In other words, we end up prioritizing the rush of indulging in tempting foods and ditching our healthy intentions because we fail to imagine and identify with our hoped-for selves. You can see how this contributes to the intention-action gap, making it more difficult to achieve the results you crave. This near-sighted tendency is well documented, especially when it comes to the challenge of saving for the future. In a 2009 study published in the journal *Social Cognitive and Affective Neuroscience*, psychologist Hal Hershfield examined people's willingness to give up immediate monetary rewards in favor of a larger but delayed payoff, but get this: There wasn't much difference between the way people thought about their future selves and the way they thought about *complete strangers*. Not surprisingly, this disconnect made them less concerned with cashing in on a reward they'd have to wait for. Interestingly, though, in a groundbreaking follow-up series of studies published in a 2011 issue of the *Journal of Marketing Research*, Hershfield found that when participants interacted with virtual renderings of their older selves via virtual reality, they were much more likely to engage in behaviors—such as giving greater weight to long-term saving—that would benefit themselves in years to come. These studies were all about trading present financial gains for larger payoffs down the line, but if you're wondering why we're suddenly talking about 401k's, the same principles apply to other types of behavior (*especially* eating).

To put this in perspective: Many of us are so fixated on what we want right now that we end up treating our future selves like *total randos*. We eat past-their-prime baked goods and rummage our pantries late-night without a second thought, because without a clear connection to our healthy future selves, it's extra challenging to resist immediate food impulses. But we've got to stop treating the future versions of us like strangers, because the research suggests that the more actively people think about their later selves, the less likely they are to say "screw it" to their long-term goals, whether they're financial *or* health-related.

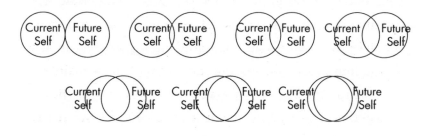

As Hershfield's research demonstrates, when you start thinking about your eventual self as an extension of your current self, it's a lot easier to make decisions in the here-and-now that are in line with what you want for yourself later on (think of it as doing your eventual self a solid). For example, when you come home from a late night out, conjuring thoughts of your future self (even your *tomorrow-morning self*) can encourage you to chug water and call it a night, rather than raiding the fridge or pantry. Instead of defaulting to a picked-over pastry during a snoozefest of a meeting, you might choose to slowly sip your coffee for the sake of helping out the forthcoming version of you.

One of the best examples of this is what I like to call the bridal phenomenon. I love working with brides because they always *kill it*: In my experience, brides are the most focused, steadfast, in-it-to-win-it clients around, and that's because making healthy changes doesn't feel like some arbitrary goal; since they can *imagine* (often with great specificity) what consistent, healthy changes will look and feel like, they're much less conflicted about fleeting temptations. Brides-to-be can envision their future selves reaping the benefits of their hard work: slipping on that stunning dress and walking with confidence down the aisle. Whether you care about weddings and white dresses or not, let me tell you, that's powerful stuff.

If you've ever made some real get-healthy progress in the past, you know how much more motivating it is to maintain healthy-eating tweaks after you've already made some headway (whether that's going down a jean size, feeling sexier naked, or having more energy or more vibrant skin). After getting a small taste of how good progress feels, it's easier to keep honoring those adjustments and turning them into enduring habits. When you can literally *see* and *feel* the results of your efforts, it's less of a stretch to imagine how great you might feel six months or a year from now—a major source of encouragement to keep on keeping on.

GETTING TO KNOW THE FUTURE YOU

I know, *I know*: It's not always so easy to envision a future version of yourself in the abstract. The first step is to hone in on what you really want for yourself down the line, so you can get to work translating your intentions into concrete actions. To kick off the process, give this exercise a try and see what images come to mind:

Close your eyes and picture the best possible version of yourself next year. You're still you in all the ways that make you unique, but it's a year later and you've worked through many of your get-healthy challenges, and quite frankly, you're *thriving*. Zoom in on this image: How do you feel? More specifically, how would you want this best-possible, next-year version of you to feel? (The more vividly you can envision yourself this way, the better...so get detailed.) How do you want to feel when you get out of bed? When you take a shower, moisturize your bod, and then slip on your clothes?

How about when you walk into work? When you stand, exercise, have sex? Are you moving through the day with energy and confidence? Go ahead and close your eyes, I'll wait...

Also, think about the future perks of executing your get-healthy goals: What would you like to be able to *do* physically next year or the following year? Many of us tend to fixate on a particular occasion—the way we'd like to look at a big event or on vacation. That's all fine, but these are extrinsic benchmarks, so they don't hold a lot of weight after the occasion has passed. A more effective approach is to envision the lasting benefits of your hard work and what's in it for *you*—whether it's having more energy, clearer, dewier skin, or a greater sense of comfort in your body, being able to dance longer or hike faster...you get the point. Imagining these possibilities makes your future-self dynamic—a true extension of you—so you're less inclined to dismiss your next-year goals when you're faced with the lure of an instantly gratifying treat. Like my brides discovered, the more closely you can connect to yourself in the future, the less conflicted you'll feel about eating in ways that will help you attain *and maintain* your big-picture goals.

Our day-to-day relationship with food involves balancing the tradeoffs between our long-term pursuits and immediate wants, which are often in conflict. For example, most people want to look and feel better—they want to feel more confident, more vibrant, have more energy—and, at the same time, they also want the donut at the staff meeting and an extra serving of pasta at book club. But I want to make one thing crystal clear: Having a healthy relationship with food *doesn't* mean always choosing the eating behavior that supports the long-lens goal over the immediate want (because, let's be real, that sounds like a total drag). Instead, it's about having the ability to pause and consider the options at hand and then make a conscious choice. For example: *Do I really want this donut?* If the answer is yes, then put it on a plate, enjoy it slowly, and then move on *without* stressing about the freaking donut for the rest of the day. In the next chapter you'll learn specific techniques to help you get there.

TREAT YO SELF VS. TREAT YO FUTURE SELF

All too often we accept the deadbeat booty call even when we're ready to settle down, because we can't actually imagine ourselves finding the love of our lives. The same pattern happens with food, meaning it's much easier to say f-it to our long-term health goals if we can't actually connect with the person who will be enjoying the eventual perks down the road. So, in order to balance the pursuit of your high-altitude aspirations with your immediate desires, it's crucial to have a clear and realistic vision for how you want to be in six months, next year, or five years from now. Then you can start investing in your future self by acting in ways that reconcile your current and long-term wishes. To close that gap, start imagining your future self reaping the benefits of a healthy relationship with food. Imagine how liberating it will feel to really enjoy what you eat, guilt- and drama-free. Think of all the headspace and energy you'll save that you could devote to other stuff. Consider how good you'll feel in your own skin, without being at war with yourself over your food choices. If you tap into that future sense of satisfaction, it will help pull you further toward making thoughtful food choices today for a healthier tomorrow. When you make food choices from this place of clarity and focus, *you're* in charge, so you're in a better position to push back against the forces (in your head *and* your environment) that could throw you off course.

The takeaway: Being able to vividly picture and relate to a realistic version of yourself in the future can help you carry out behaviors now that will facilitate more valuable payoffs to come. In a pair of studies, published in the June 2013 issue of *Psychological Science*, researchers found that when people strengthened their ability to distinctly imagine their future selves by writing a letter to their older selves, they were less inclined to make "delinquent" choices (like buying potentially stolen stuff or committing insurance fraud); what's more, after they interacted with realistically aged, digitized versions of themselves, they were less likely to cheat on a subsequent trivia test. Long story short, imagining a detailed version of yourself in the future can enhance your capacity to pass up the immediate satisfaction of acting impulsively on fleeting food cravings, in favor of long-term payoffs. If you're a parent or you'd like to be a parent someday, another helpful way to connect to the future is to imagine yourself adopting one of the healthy-eating habits you've been struggling with and then picture your children or future children embracing that habit, too. For many of us, prioritizing our kids' (even our unborn kids') futures can help shift the stakes and encourage us to reevaluate the way we think about tempting food choices in the present.

One of the best techniques for harnessing this connectedness with the future is to write a letter to the eventual you, which may sound ridiculous, but can be surprisingly effective (if you don't BS or wing it). If what you write is personal and meaningful to you, the letter can give you some serious clarity about what you really want, what your goals are, and how you'd like to conduct yourself, look, and feel in the not-too-distant future (maybe one, two, or five years down the line). To put yourself in the right frame of mind, I like to take this activity a step further and make it a letter of gratitude to your future self, one in which you acknowledge the efforts it took to become a healthier *you,* and thank yourself for making that happen.

To get the process started, think about the following:

What would it feel like to see your healthy future self in action?

What kinds of food-related obstacles do you face now that you want to conquer?

What get-healthy goals do you aspire to achieve?

How would you like to feel, look, and move in your own bod?

What would you want to be able to say to that super-healthy version of you?

NOW WHAT?

Once you have a vision of your future self a year or more from now, it's time to pay yourself forward with your eating behavior. Make a list of some of the goals you would like to achieve, then map out some actionable strategies for how you might get there. For instance, if you want to make more conscious decisions about what you eat, framing this as "becoming more mindful" is too vague to be effective; a better approach is to think about what you can do to set yourself up to make more conscious eating decisions on the regular, whether it's by building in a pause before you reach for something to nibble on, or prepping healthy snacks ahead of time.

To come up with these pay-yourself-forward strategies, be prepared to make *some* compromises for the sake of your future self. Yes, eating *should* be enjoyable, but it's not possible to cater to your every right-now craving and still get the future outcome you desire. *I know that you already know that.* But that said, this doesn't mean you have to choose the berries over the baked goods every time, either.

It's a matter of balancing your food choices, weighing the relative benefits and tradeoffs of going one way or another, and reconciling conflicting desires (which we all have, btw).

For example, maybe *you want to prep healthy snacks for the week over the weekend,* but *you also want to maximize your weekend lounge time.* Or *perhaps you want to eat more healthfully at restaurants* but *you also want to fully enjoy what you order when dining out.* These examples illustrate common conflicting desires at play. *What to do?* The first step is to question whether the conflicting desires are really mutually exclusive. Could you spend a few minutes prepping healthy snacks for the week and still maximize your weekend lounge time? (*Definitely*, especially if you're efficient in the kitchen, or if you opt to buy prewashed and precut veggies.) Does eating more healthfully at restaurants mean you can't fully enjoy what you're having? (*No.* It's a matter of deciding what's worth splurging on and what's not.)

Looking at conflicting desires this way when it comes to food helps illuminate areas where you can find a middle ground, and others where you may need to get real with yourself. Take a moment to make a list of what you perceive to be your own conflicting desires, then consider whether they really do exclude each other, whether there's an opportunity for give-and-take, or—assuming your endgame is of great importance to you—whether you need to reprioritize. In some cases, you don't actually have to make a choice: For example, you could hang with friends and cook a healthy meal together, an arrangement that makes it possible to fully enjoy your eating experience without abandoning your get-healthy intentions *or* your good times.

GIVING YOUR GOALS A REALITY CHECK

It's also important to weed out disingenuous goals. This is partly about making changes for the right reasons (because *you* want to, not because your mother or partner wants you to, or because you think that's what everyone else is doing). So consider: Are your wellness ambitions intended to help you achieve *your* best possible self or Gisele's? It may seem like an absurd question, but you'd be surprised how many people point to pictures on their phones of *other* (often photoshopped) people when I ask them to tell me what their goals are. This doesn't work, because no matter how motivated you are, eating more healthfully will *not* change how tall you are or your bone structure. Accepting this is crucial.

One of the most moving moments in my career was when a then-14-year-old client described this acceptance perfectly. She was a whip-smart young lady, about 5'2", attending a competitive all-girls high school, and she matter-of-factly declared, "All my best friends are 5'10" and blonde and can virtually eat whatever they want, and you know what? Of course, I wish I could eat that way, but I can't, so I'd like to learn how to eat for me." We talked about what a balanced day of eating looks like and how to arm herself with healthy (but still delish) school snacks so she wouldn't be tempted by the treat du jour unless it was something she really fancied (like macarons or mini cupcakes). I still get a little choked up thinking about her, because her perspective was so evolved, and (unfortunately) *so uncommon*. This girl is undoubtedly going places.

Along the way, it's important to suss out whether your goals are realistic. Ask yourself: Do my get-healthy aspirations leave room for flexibility? Are they attainable given what I'm doing now? Often people throw down blanket declarations like "I'm quitting sugar," but this can be a real challenge because the statement is so all-encompassing and doesn't distinguish between natural sugars or added sugars. If someone takes a hard-line approach to this goal, it means ditching fruit and healthful complex carbs (like sweet potatoes), not to mention banning birthday cake. If you'd prefer not to eat birthday cake ever again, that's cool with me, but don't feel like you *need* to be ultra-extreme in order to reach your target. Instead, I usually recommend a far more reasonable and humane approach, like aiming to avoid *added* sugar (in beverages, salad dressings, nut butters, and so on) while still giving yourself the option to have some sugar in moderation (even birthday cake).

Also, consider: Are you motivated to get healthier or lose weight because you believe that by doing so everything else in your life will suddenly fall into place? (That's not a legit goal.) On the other hand, if you're motivated to make lifestyle changes because you want to feel more confident, have more energy, and be a leaner, stronger, healthier version of *yourself*, you're headed in the right direction. Another common goal-setting glitch: aiming for the stars when you can barely get off the ground because of time constraints. I talk to so many clients who have incredibly jam-packed schedules— whether it's due to school, work, home, other obligations, or some combination thereof—and as much as they wish they could make Pinterest-worthy dinners on the regular, that's just not realistic for them; so they end up feeling like failures when they're unable to execute their good intentions.

Here's the thing: It's fine if you can cook only once a week (or not at all), as long as you're honest with yourself about that. Once you let go of false promises, you can invest your efforts in legit solutions, like doctoring up a good-quality store-bought rotisserie chicken and making healthy assembly-only side dishes to go with it (see Part Two). Be honest with yourself about what you can realistically pull off, then identify and ditch those unrealistic goals you've been hanging onto. You'll be thrilled with how liberating this feels.

Remember: You want to be able to feel great now as well as in the future, so the goal for today is to make healthy, balanced, flexible food choices that are sustainable for the long haul. The point isn't to set yourself up for a spartan lifestyle that's rich in self-denial. What you're trying to do here is make lasting changes to your eating patterns that will become healthy habits *for life*. To keep honoring that commitment day after day, you'll need to lean in and stay focused and connected to yourself for both the present and future; the next chapter will help you get there.

4

Tune In to Your True Desires

Be honest: Have you ever been on the phone with your loved one and been called out for not really listening? Maybe the tip-off was a couple of misplaced *yeahs* or *uh-huhs*, or maybe the other person could hear the clack of keystrokes on a computer? I think we can all agree that this scenario feels pretty messed up when you're on the receiving end. And yet, employing communication strategies like these in the name of efficiency is certainly not uncommon. Sure, we're all busy and we're encouraged to multitask like jugglers on unicycles, but *really* listening is not something we can afford to ditch (in our love lives *or* our eating lives).

Any relationship expert (or daytime talk-show host) will tell you that getting good at listening is key when it comes to staying connected *and* staying out of the doghouse. That's because being fully present and engaged offers something incredibly valuable: a real understanding of what's going on beneath your partner's surface, so you can respond accordingly and avoid misunderstandings. Staying up to date on your S.O.'s inner world can definitely feel like an impossible task if your focus is elsewhere, but there's a lot less static when you tune in and keep your antenna up. Our relationship with food and our bodies is no different.

In the same way that leaning in and actively listening to your significant other helps you better understand them, focusing on your body's signals can help you distinguish between legit physiological hunger and simply feeling peckish, or between feeling satisfied and overly stuffed. So let's become better listeners—by paying attention to those subtle internal cues that we're all so used to ignoring. The typical advice, *Eat when you're hungry, stop when you're full*, isn't misguided, but the reality is not quite that simple. Because, for instance, *what if you're not really sure?* Most people aren't.

Feeling comfortably full after eating is certainly the goal, but since hunger and satiety cues can be so vague and elusive, getting to the right place doesn't always feel like a breeze. No worries if you don't actually know what being comfortably full feels like—that's totally fine (and very common). *I promise you.* A good place to start is to think about a sensation I imagine just about everyone *has* experienced: feeling *uncomfortably* full. Can you recall a time when you felt overstuffed? No need to dwell on any disappointment or stress that came with the overeating episode; simply focus on the physical sensation of being stuffed beyond reason. Unpleasant, right? Something you'd like to avoid in the future, yes? As you discovered in Chapter 3, calling on personal experiences (imagined and otherwise) can help guide your eating behavior in any given moment. Let's say you're really digging a meal, and you realize you're approaching capacity but you want to keep eating anyway—it can be helpful to nonjudgmentally recall a time when an otherwise enjoyable eating experience morphed into a not-so-comfy one. Summoning up the way your stomach felt distended like an overcommitted suitcase, and perhaps how sluggish you felt afterward, can help you pump the brakes when you're approaching satiety and avoid burdening yourself with a bellyache.

Trust me on this, because I've been there. A few years ago, my husband and I went to an incredible anniversary dinner at a really special Italian restaurant in New York City called Babbo. We had received a generous gift certificate for our wedding, but given our schedules and the insane (but understandable) reservation waiting list, we ended up going a year later. My husband was determined to use the entire gift certificate to avoid the hassle of rebooking, and in doing so, he ordered just about everything on the menu "to try." But since all the dishes were unquestionably next-level delicious, he had trouble holding back and went a bit overboard. To be honest, I did, too, and we spent the night in sweats, downing ginger tea and Googling alternative gas and heartburn remedies... not exactly the romantic night we had in mind. Thankfully, we both laughed about it then, and it's something we still joke about to this day, but the memory also lives on as a reminder *not* to pull a Babbo (no matter how next-level the menu is).

Finding your comfortably full zone is a supremely

individualized experience, but assuming you've felt the sensations of being overstuffed and physiologically hungry, you know that the sweet spot is somewhere between the two ends of the spectrum. You want to feel satisfied, but without having to unbutton or unzip your jeans. Getting to that optimal place consistently is something that will get a lot easier once you make a real effort to locate it...knowing that there *will* be times when you overshoot and feel *too* full, and also times when you think you're full and then 30 minutes later you feel legitimately hungry again. It's up to you to honor that signal your body is giving you and make sure you're not going hungry. People always ask me what's the right cutoff for eating at night. The answer is, there is no real cutoff. Nobody should go to bed hungry. What a horrible feeling!

GIVING YOUR INNER GAUGES A TUNE-UP

We all have implicit cues that help us figure out how much food we actually want and need. But as adults we can't always hear those signals because they get overridden by other influences (such as bad moods, stress, and distractions) and because our internal communication travels at the speed of dial-up, while our cravings zoom around on broadband. Complicating matters, anyone who has been on a restrictive diet (as many people have) has repeatedly told the brain not to listen to the body in the face of true physiological hunger;

it's as if you've practiced ghosting those internal cues. (Not to worry: You *can* change this.)

Since ignoring your body's hunger and comfortably full cues isn't exactly in your best interest, it's time to reverse this tendency. The key is to harness the power of your prefrontal cortex (PFC), the part of the brain that's like command central for self-awareness and willpower. Think of it as the control panel that helps you resist instantly gratifying behaviors in favor of bigger payoffs for your future self. The PFC is the part of the brain that helps you break out of your Netflix binge and go to the gym instead because the latter offers more long-term benefits. Or forgo the decadent chocolate sundae at a restaurant in favor of the dark chocolate you have waiting for you at home because the latter is more in line with achieving your long-term get-healthy goals.

If you imagine the different parts of your brain as a group of friends with *very* different personalities, maturity levels, and values, the PFC would be the sage, uber-reasonable diplomat of the bunch. When you encounter an appealing stimulus—such as a giant piece of chocolate cake—all the friends perk up and weigh in on what to do next. Most of the pals are interested in doubling down on pleasure, and they aren't shy about letting the PFC know where they stand on the cake ("Go for it!," "*Need!*," "Eat it NOW."). But when the PFC is actively engaged, it's able to weigh the relative pros and cons of having the cake (or not) and make a solid, thoughtful decision for the group. So, if the PFC ultimately decides that while the huge wedge of chocolate cake *does* look and smell *incredible*, you're not actually dying for it, so you'll pass *this* time; or perhaps, after mulling it over, the PFC may decide that you would in fact love to have a sliver, on a plate, so that you can savor every morsel. There is no right answer here. Both are valid choices, because they're both thoughtful ones.

If you've had trouble making food-related decisions this way in the past, you may be wondering: If the PFC is supposed to be so good at weighing our right-now wants against our long-term goals and making consciously healthy food choices, is mine straight-up broken? No, but it is *perpetually distracted*. It's true that your PFC is your greatest ally when it comes to making conscious food choices and resisting the urge to overeat or jump at every baked good you see; the only wrinkle is that the PFC is extra vulnerable to stress and distractions. When your attention is all over the place or you're stressed out or painfully self-critical, for instance, your PFC essentially checks out and leaves the decision-making to its more impulsive (*present-biased*) brain-dwelling cohorts, which quite frankly couldn't care less about the future or your get-healthy goals. This hopefully explains why you (or anyone else) could be totally motivated to eat a certain way and yet still not follow through, because you're literally surrounded by distractions and your PFC ends up MIA.

Between the ever-growing list of modern-day distractions—e-mail, texts, apps, social media alerts—the PFC is often too frazzled to help us make the best food choices. As you're well aware, we're constantly asking our brains to shift attention from one task or screen to another. All of this multitasking ramps up production of the stress hormone cortisol, which can contribute to impulsivity and lead us to make food choices that aren't in line with our get-healthy goals. It's a lousy cycle because the more distracted and stressed we are, the less self-awareness we have, which makes it even harder to listen to the internal signals that are supposed to be guiding our eating behavior—and easier to slip into a feeding frenzy.

Plus, eating is a seriously multisensory act, so when your focus isn't on the meal you're eating, it's easy to lose touch with how you're feeling. It's almost as if the eating experience doesn't fully register. Case in point: A study at the University of Birmingham in the UK found that when young women watched TV while they ate lunch, they ate significantly more cookies during their subsequent afternoon snack than their peers who didn't watch TV. As the researchers noted in a 2009 issue of *Appetite*, watching television while eating prevented the women from fully enjoying the sensory properties of the food they were eating and properly encoding the memory of the meal. (It's almost as if they had a mild case of eating amnesia.) Spoiler alert: The same thing can happen if you're scrolling through social media feeds while you're eating.

As we know, most of us struggle with these distractions on a daily basis. Our brains are busier than ever. And since the ubiquity of daily stressors and digital technology isn't going away, we need to focus on ways to tune in to ourselves (our moods, our feelings, what our bodies are telling us) and really focus on eating *while eating* despite these challenges. I'm all for keeping things efficient, but when it comes to eating, multitasking is a great way to ensure that your PFC is out to lunch. I get it—I'm a realist—and sometimes you simply *have* to eat at your computer because you're crunched for time (same here). But in those times, you need to be willing to say to yourself that since you are distracted while eating, it's likely that you could finish your entire meal and not really process that it happened; keep this reality in mind when you lunge for a snack 15 minutes later, too.

The truth is, when it comes to making healthy food choices consistently, it's all about focusing on the most important *yet* often overlooked factor in the eating equation: the brain. The more vividly you process your food experiences and the more attuned you are to your body's signals, the more adept you'll be at making *intentional* food choices. This is where your PFC becomes your BFF: If you take steps to engage your PFC, you're less likely to be thrown off course in the face of triggers (like stress and distractions)—even when you're tired, sad, or *over* everything. It's scientifically proven that each of us can rewire our brains and improve our ability to harness the PFC just like we can strengthen the muscles in our body—through practice, practice, and more of the same.

THE WANT-IT BALANCING ACT

Quite simply, comparing short-term desires (hello, sugar cravings) against big-picture wellness goals (like looking and feeling your best next year) requires a great deal of focus and attention—especially in the PFC. The trouble is, even periodic bouts of intense stress can really impede functioning in this area. This is why office dwellers often end up hitting the communal pantry for stale-ish pretzels (even if they don't even really like pretzels to begin with) when their jam-packed inboxes seem insurmountable. Thankfully, it's possible to adapt our response to these types of stressors, giving us more flexibility and perspective when life isn't going according to plan (as it rarely does).

Consider one of my clients who couldn't stop overeating. Lily, an artist, often spent her days buried in her work and late nights at art shows; when she popped up for air she'd binge on fast food, pizza, ramen, you name it. The interesting thing was that she was very deliberate and precise about her work and the way she sourced her materials. So much care and effort and thought went into every single detail—her work was a huge source of pride.

While we were working together, it became clear that she thought about her materials and her art the same way I like to think about food and the body. I think it's much easier to eat with awareness and intention if the food you're eating feels special. For instance, if you go to a farmers' market, it's kind of impossible not to notice that for the individuals who grow, harvest, or catch the food, that's not just their job, it's their *craft*. I'd argue that most legit farmers aren't ripping food out of the ground and tossing it into boxes willy-nilly (after all, the produce would look pretty funky in that case); they are gentle and purposeful in the same way my client was when she sought out materials for her artwork. We talked about shifting her mindset this way, and it was like a light bulb went on for her. The good news was that she was already purposeful in one area of her life; she just had to practice using that same focus with eating. Lily started going to the farmers' market and getting inspired by the colors, tastes, and textures. Thinking about food choices in a more curated way—which required harnessing her PFC—helped Lily eat more thoughtfully and in turn get a handle on her previously chaotic eating habits.

PUTTING YOUR PFC TO GOOD USE

Unlike muscles, your PFC doesn't need endless reps and intervals to be strengthened. It thrives on intentional use, enough good sleep, and positive emotions. One thing we know for sure is that slowing down helps engage the PFC on an everyday basis—and no, you don't have to move to an ashram to do it. Taking your time and focusing on moment-to-moment experiences with food also improves self-control and lets you hit the brakes on autopilot behavior, which is why you can't go anywhere without hearing someone wax poetic about the benefits of mindfulness. Not interested in becoming a monk? Me, neither. At this point, simply telling someone to eat more *mindfully* usually elicits (and warrants) eye-rolling. People *know* they should be more focused while they're eating, but many just don't know *how* to make the shift. So I began recommending techniques to help remedy that.

Think about it: How freaking good does it feel when all of

your senses are engaged in romantic situations when you're totally in the moment and savoring every little detail? You want to do the same thing with your food—well, maybe not the *same* thing, but you know what I mean. Eating isn't just about taste; it's also about touch, smell, sight, and sound. Here are practical ways you can tune in to the full sensory experience of eating and make more fully engaged choices— without all the New Age jargon.

Swap hands: This can feel awkward at first but the perk is that eating with your nondominant hand forces you to concentrate harder on eating *while* eating. The process interrupts the habit of eating sans body awareness, giving you more control over what you actually put into your mouth. Another helpful tactic: putting your fork down between bites; it builds in a pause that lets you reassess your hunger.

Take a hands-on approach: There's no question that ditching the utensil middleman helps focus your attention on eating. Using your hands allows you to experience the physical sensation of eating even before the food hits your mouth. (It probably goes without saying, but just to be clear: It's best to reserve this practice for solid foods and nonjudgmental company.)

Plating matters: Would you serve your crush a meal out of a soggy take-out container? *Exactly.* Whether you're dining solo or with company, make sure it's done with some level of dignity (i.e., on a plate). Being able to visualize what and how much you're eating is an important part of the eating-awareness process. Many of us go all editorial with food presentation when serving a meal to our partners, families, friends (and Instagram community), but end up eating hurriedly over the sink when it's just us. But when food is plated it makes the process feel real and substantial, and it also helps prevent overeating. I'm not saying go full Cordon Bleu, but do yourself a favor and put what you're going to eat on a plate.

Turn up the lights: Mood lighting is lovely, but it can disconnect you from what you're eating. Make sure you can see what's on your plate so you stay in touch with what and how much you're consuming. Similarly, regardless of how sweet your sound system is, keep your background music at a reasonable volume so you don't give yourself another form of sensory overload that will distract you from the pleasure of eating or speed up your intake.

Get sensual: Before you tuck into a meal, savor the aromas. While you're eating, notice every taste and texture, even the subtle ones; focus on how the food feels in your mouth and as it gently slips down your throat. Besides giving you more pleasure from your meal, slowing down while eating also gives your brain time to catch up with your gut and register the presence of food. This can help you eat enough so that you're comfortably full, but not so much that you feel like you're expectant with a full-term food baby. In fact, a 2011 study in the journal *Appetite* revealed that when consumers are asked to focus on what they're eating in terms of how they'd rank the pleasantness of the taste and their desire to continue eating that particular food, that focus actually reduces their intake compared to when they think about different foods or something else entirely. Chewing longer can also help in this respect by allowing you to savor the flavors. Plus, it enhances meal memory, which is a good thing because when a meal is memorable and pleasurable, you're less likely to overeat later on.

Stop stealing food: Have you ever taken sneaky bites out of a pie box in the fridge or on the counter and told yourself they didn't count? The reality is, most of those bites add up to a small sliver (or more), except you didn't get to enjoy that piece because it was parceled into stealthy bites that you were trying not to acknowledge. Better to be up front and serve yourself what you want on a plate (see above) so that it becomes a legit eating experience you can fully enjoy. The same is true when it comes to eating from a bag or a box: Put the chips or nuts or chocolate on a plate or little dish (even a shot glass). Own the noshing session and savor it; this way, you'll avoid the mindless hand-to-mouth moves that come from eating out of a package.

Gauge your hunger with crudités: I figured this one out when I was in grad school. Quite stressed, without much structure to my days, I ended up snacking all day and losing touch with my hunger cues, and then being kind of dissatisfied with dinner because I had been snacking all day. As I discovered, one easy way to gauge hunger is by keeping fresh crudités (raw veggies like carrots, cucumbers, and bell peppers, that have been washed and cut) and a tasty dip at eye level in the fridge at all times. If you're between meals or post-snack but you're not totally satisfied, go for the crudités. If you don't want the crudités, you're probably not really hungry. In my practice, I see a lot of students, moms, freelancers, actors, and other people who don't have much built-in structure to their days often grab for snacks when they're stressed or procrastinating—they, too, have found that the crudités trick really works!

Abandon stale mindsets: First of all, kick guilt about wasting food and the need to clean your plate to the curb. Those notions really don't help anyone—besides, *hello? Leftovers.* Similarly, be willing to abort a food mission if it's not satisfying you. I have an amazingly sassy and direct friend who straight-up terminates dates midway if they aren't going well. She's polite about it, but she's busy and her free time is scarce, and if she can tell the vibe isn't working, she politely and respectfully pulls the escape hatch (in case you're wondering, her suitors usually respect and appreciate her transparency). I feel the same way about food—there's no reason to force something that you *know* isn't working. If you're not enjoying a particular food, put it down. Just like there's no point in spending an evening trudging through a meh date, there's no reason to keep eating a meh food.

GETTING INTO THE RIGHT EATING GROOVE

If you want to start eating with all your senses perked up, pay attention to your body *before* you put food in your mouth.

Step 1: Assess your body sensations.

How do you feel overall right this very moment? Relaxed? Stressed? Distracted? Sleepy? Bored? Are any areas of your body particularly tight? Next, rate your hunger: On a scale from that post-Thanksgiving *stuffed* feeling to you could eat anything in sight, how hungry are you? Did your hunger come on quickly, or was it more of a slow roll? Is your stomach rumbling? Is your mouth watering?

Step 2: Serve yourself a meal or snack.

(This assumes you're dealing with legit hunger.) Then, ask yourself the following before you eat it:

- What does the food smell like? Does it bring any specific food memories to mind?
- What does the food look like? Are the colors bright or muted? What about the texture?
- If it's hot, can you see the steam rising?
- What does it sound like when you lower your fork, spoon, or knife into it or pick it up with your hands? Do you have to break it apart first? Can you sense anything more specific about the texture? Is it warm or cold to the touch?

(continued on next page)

Step 3: Place the first bite in your mouth.

Now, consider:

- Is it warm or cold when it arrives in your mouth?
- Is it light and airy? Dense or slippery?
- Is it bitter or sweet? Savory or salty?
- How is the initial flavor working out for you? Is it worthy of your taste buds? If you're not loving the taste, and you're in a position to switch gears, are you open to finding a better option you'll enjoy more?
- If it's a dish you haven't had before, try to identify the specific flavors, herbs, and spices. What pops out to you?
- If it's something you've had before, how does the taste compare to the last time you had it? If you were to make the dish in the future, is there anything you would tweak? Would you make it spicier? Saltier? Less sweet?

Step 4: Continue eating.

Make a concerted effort to truly taste every bite. When you think you're about 25 percent done eating, put down your utensils, pause, and check in with yourself again:

- Consider whether you've detected any more subtle flavors or taste sensations.
- Think about how the food felt in your mouth and as it traveled to your stomach.

- Speaking of, how is your stomach feeling *now*? Are you feeling less hungry or more satisfied? Does sipping water affect your hunger?

Resume eating and ask yourself these questions again when you think you're 50 percent through the meal and again at 75 percent.

Step 5: Scan your body when you finish eating.

Ask yourself:

- Do I feel satisfied?
- Am I still slightly hungry?
- Did I overshoot it?

Zero judgment here! The point is to simply pay attention to eating *while* eating and how you're feeling so you can adjust your approach in the future.

What you're doing with these exercises is wrangling the PFC in order to help you tune out all the white noise and make intentional eating choices. Once you begin taking steps to keep tuning in to yourself in the face of distractions, you'll be less vulnerable to the obstacles presented by the modern world. Most importantly, these strategies were designed with reality in mind. I realize that there will be times when you'll need to eat in front of your laptop, or while tending to rambunctious children, because, hey, that's real life. Staying attuned to what you're doing and how you're feeling will help you navigate these unruly moments with greater ease and comfort. The practice will also help you pause and consider what you really want to eat and what's realistic in any given situation.

In the next chapter, you'll discover strategies that will make it easier to achieve this without overtaxing your PFC. That's not to say there won't be times when you overdo it and eat until you're excessively stuffed (*ahem*, Babbo). But the more attention you pay to your body's cues, the easier it will be to make choices that, more often than not, serve your long-term interests as well as your immediate wants. With this approach, you'll be well on your way to establishing the kind of relationship with food I think everyone is after: healthier and more respectful, but still lusty and passionate.

5

Take the Pressure Off

You know those times (past or present) when you give your friend your cell phone at the beginning of a night out because you don't trust yourself to not text your ex? It's pretty genius, actually. First, you had the foresight and self-awareness to recognize that you might be in a particularly vulnerable state of mind later on. You essentially precommitted to acting in your own best interest. This way, in a moment of weakness, you didn't even have the option to act in a way that wasn't in line with your more rational plans for yourself. The decision was already made for you (and even better, *by* you).

When it comes to eating decisions, altering your world in ways that make it easier to act in your own best interest works the same way (read: really well). Why? As you're well aware, overriding real-time impulses and desires in order to make food choices that reflect your big-picture, get-healthy goals isn't always a cinch. It takes *a lot* of focus. As you saw in the last chapter, honing your willpower skills and paying attention to your body's internal cues while you're eating is crucial to improving your noshing habits. But where people often go amiss is relying *exclusively* on willpower, because it isn't always available to us.

Research suggests that any time we're wielding deliberate control over our behavior, we're drawing from the same willpower well. This concept applies whether you're opting to slow your eating when you're approaching capacity (despite wanting to keep going), trying to get to class or work on time (when you'd rather be snoozing), refraining from epic spending sprees, resisting the urge to roll your eyes at people who annoy you—the list goes on. The trouble is, once our willpower reserves are empty, we're much more likely to make impulsive decisions that aren't consistent with our intentions and what we really want. *Not ideal.*

Think of the times when you've come home after a grueling day with every intention of whipping up (or ordering) a healthy meal, only to find yourself grabbing something quick from your pantry. Or the times you've put off a morning workout and told yourself you'd exercise later in the afternoon, but ultimately excused yourself because you felt drained from your jam-packed day. We've all been there. They're prime examples of willpower depletion in action, when you've relied on self-control so heavily that it kind of maxes out, and now you can't capably deal. In 2008, a team of researchers, led by Kathleen Vohs, found that it isn't just exerting self-control that drains willpower—excessive decision-making does, too. Hence, the term *decision fatigue*, which explains why we tend to default to something noncommittal like crackers and hummus when we've spun our wheels trying to figure out what to eat for dinner, why we buy unnecessary things in checkout lines after big shopping hauls, and why we opt for warranties we don't really need—because (consciously or not) we're thinking, *Enough with the decisions already!*

The information-overload world (yet again) poses some serious challenges in this department. Just think of all the mini-decisions posed by looking at your Facebook newsfeed for all of five minutes—whether to send an absurd meme to a friend (and if so, by FB Messenger, e-mail, or text?), watch the video everyone is buzzing about, buy the pants FB somehow knows you considered purchasing last week, wish your acquaintance a happy birthday, or get back to work. Basically, our brains were designed to handle only so many decisions and so much data in a day, so when we're overly inundated with choices, it's like withdrawing willpower cash as if we have unlimited funds, and we end up without much self-control toward the middle and end of the day. When you think about it, how could it be any other way? Get this: It's estimated that we have 300 exabytes (that's 300,000,000,000,000,000,000 pieces!) of human-created information available at our fingertips at all times, according to behavioral neuroscientist Daniel Levitin, author of *The Organized Mind*. That's *a lot* of data and mundane choices to sort through, and as a result, our minds are often too fatigued to decide what's best for us to eat. Even for the most rational Type-A personalities among us, our capacity for willpower is limited and can become depleted with overuse, just like an overworked muscle can if you were to do endless push-ups or planks. But unlike being physically spent, where there are telltale signs like shaky muscles and achy joints, willpower fatigue isn't that easy to spot. So we continue on with our days, making choice after choice, trying to exert self-control, and eventually we end up acting impulsively or simply relinquishing control altogether ("I don't care—just order for me!").

Not all is lost. There are ways to conserve your willpower— and it's easier than you may think (no heavy lifting required). In fact, the more structure you provide in your day-to-day life, the less self-control you actually need to close the gap between your good eating intentions and effective everyday actions. This approach seriously simplifies the what-to-eat equation and limits the number of food-related decisions you'll need to make throughout the day. Doing so helps you save your willpower reserve for times when you *really* need it (post-breakup, mid-work disaster, when young children are wailing). To make this happen, it's wise to engage in some precommitment: Map out how you want to behave ahead of time in order to limit the likelihood of acting impulsively in the heat of the moment. People who rely on precommitment know that it works, but recently researchers have revealed *how*. Remember the prefrontal cortex (the PFC), the super-rational part of the brain that helps us make thoughtful, future-oriented food choices? Well, a study published in *Neuron* found that when people engage in precommitment in the face of temptations, there's more connectivity between the areas of the brain involved in decision-making and the PFC, making impulsivity less likely.

To tame the lure of immediate temptations, you can pre-commit to solid decisions in many different ways. For example, if you're planning to order in for dinner, do so *before* you leave the office or wherever you are, rather than after you get home. The hungrier you are when you're ordering, the more impulsive you're predisposed to be with your food choices (this is the same reason it's not the best plan to go grocery shopping when you're ravenous). By preordering, you'll be taking a preemptive strike against the impulsivity risk, and since the food will arrive when you do (or shortly thereafter), you won't have time to raid the pantry before your meal. Plus, since you already paid for the meal, you'll be less inclined to switch gears to less healthy fare. To be honest, I think this is why when friends and family members ask for my nutrition advice, they aren't usually as motivated to follow through as my clients who pay for my services are. It's the same dynamic when you have a personal trainer or a fancy gym membership: You're paying for it, so there's extra incentive to make your efforts count.

THE POWER OF FORETHOUGHT

Besides making some decisions ahead of time, you can preserve your willpower stamina in other ways, most notably by planning ahead. After all, the more straightforward you make it to follow through on your goals, the more likely you are to accomplish them. Instead of hemorrhaging self-control strength throughout the day by fighting against yourself (and the natural pull to eat tempting, instantly gratifying foods), it's far more pleasant and efficient to expend some deliberate energy on setting up game plans, habits, and rituals that will make healthy eating a no-brainer for you. Here's how to do this in different scenarios:

When dining out: If you're going out to dinner with friends and you're hoping to enjoy a delicious meal that's in line with your goals, be proactive about the kind of restaurant you choose. If you go to an Italian restaurant and you opt not to have a pasta entrée, will you feel like you're missing out? If so, suggest a different type of restaurant. Wherever you choose to go, peruse the menu beforehand so you can decide what you're going to order and what modifications you may want to ask for (for instance, subbing roasted veggies in place of a starchy side you're not that excited about, a baked sweet potato instead of fries, sweetened sauce on the side, and so on). These days, most restaurants respect it when you come in armed with specifics. So come up with yours ahead of time: This way, even if you're frazzled or stressed when it comes time to order, you'll already have a game plan ready to go. Similarly, decide ahead of time whether indulging in the restaurant's complimentary bread or chip basket is worth it to you; if not, tell your server before it gets to the table. That's one temptation down!

When eating at home: First off, start with a clean slate by going through your fridge and pantry and tossing all the expired items and stuff you just don't want to eat anymore. Now's a good time to take stock of your staples and see if added sugar has been slipped into your nut butters, sauces, and salad dressings; if it has, ditch those and replace them with ones that don't have sugar added. The next step is to set the stage for cooking healthfully at home. In order to do that, you'll want to fill your fridge and pantry with wholesome, versatile ingredients. Here are some staples to put on your grocery-shopping list:

FRIDGE ESSENTIALS

Produce: Zucchini, cauliflower, kale, romaine hearts, arugula, radicchio, cabbage, mushrooms, green beans, sugar snap peas, Brussels sprouts, carrots, avocados, bell peppers, cucumbers, sweet potatoes,* garlic,* onions,* shallots,* scallions, leeks, chile peppers, fresh thyme, fresh rosemary, fresh cilantro, fresh basil, a variety of fresh berries, dates,** lemons, limes

"Dairy" products: Unsweetened nut milk (almond, cashew, coconut, etc.), unsweetened coconut yogurt, coconut kefir, eggs

Premade items: Organic rotisserie chicken, cooked quinoa, bone broth, chicken and/or vegetable stock, precooked hardboiled eggs (optional)

Condiments that pack a serious flavor punch: Coconut aminos (a simple, healthy, umami bomb of a sauce made from aged coconut sap and sea salt), tahini, good-quality fish sauce, Dijon mustard, sauerkraut, kimchi, mayo, dairy-free pesto, hot sauce (I like Rootz and PaleoChef sriracha)

---

* Technically these can be kept in the pantry or a cool dark place.
** Whole dates should be refrigerated for maximum freshness.

Alternative flours: Coconut flour, nut flour (such as almond or hazelnut), tapioca flour, unsweetened nut butters (almond, cashew, sunflower seed)

Freezer essentials: An assortment of leafy greens (just in case), berries, cauliflower florets, green beans, and other veggies

PANTRY ESSENTIALS

Oils and vinegars: Extra-virgin olive oil, coconut oil, avocado oil, ghee, toasted sesame oil, hot sesame oil (if you like heat); apple cider vinegar, white wine vinegar, balsamic vinegar, brown rice vinegar, Champagne vinegar

Canned and bottled items: Anchovies (oil packed), salmon (oil packed), roasted tomatoes (amazing for soups and sauces), unsweetened tomato sauce, sun-dried tomatoes (oil packed), tomato paste, artichoke hearts (oil packed), olives, presoaked beans (black and chickpea), coconut milk

Spices: High-quality finishing salt, garlic powder, onion powder, toasted sesame seeds, garam masala, ground cinnamon, ground nutmeg, ground cloves, ground ginger, chili powder, ground cumin, curry powder, sumac, paprika

Miscellaneous: Nori sheets, sweet potato chips, taro root chips, kelp noodles, matcha, loose tea, a variety of raw and roasted nuts, goji berries, good-quality dark chocolate (ideally, 80 percent cacao or higher), unsweetened baking chocolate (100 percent cacao)

Staple ingredients for baking: Chia seeds, unsweetened shredded coconut, maple syrup, coconut sugar, unsweetened raw cacao powder, gluten-free vanilla extract

Semi-specialty items (but worth it): Karam's Garlic Sauce,
Majestic Garlic Spread, Trader Joe's Everything but the Bagel
seasoning, furikake (a Japanese mixed dried seasoning),
psyllium husk (a plant-based dietary fiber that works as a
powerful binder in foods), Siete Foods grain-free tortillas
and tortilla chips (available at select natural foods stores
or online)

Game-changing kitchen tools (that make life easier): A
spiralizer, a food processor, a high-speed blender such as
Vitamix, a zester, an Aerolatte frother for matcha and next-
level latte foam

SUGAR ALIASES

Generally speaking, people who go by a bunch of different
names and show up places uninvited are considered ultra-
shady, yes? Well, the same thing goes for added sugar, which
has tons of sneaky aliases and often pops up in foods and condiments where it really doesn't belong. We know it's important
to read the food labels of items we're considering taking home
from the grocery store. But that's assuming all food labels are
easy to decode. And let's be honest: Food packaging is meant
to entice us, *not* to draw our attention to added sugar.

But as long as you're on the lookout for it, you can start
to get savvy at spotting added sugar in foods—and avoiding it. The truth is, sugar is often camouflaged on ingredients
lists—as evaporated cane juice, agave, fruit juice concentrate,
brown sugar, nectar, molasses, honey, malt syrup, rice syrup,

(continued on next page)

maple syrup, corn syrup, maltodextrin, and anything ending in *ose* (dextrose, sucrose, maltose). If you see these words on an ingredients list, it means that sugar has been *added* to the product; it's not there naturally. And while some sweeteners are more healthful than others—such as minimally processed options like maple syrup, coconut sugar, and honey—it's still good to know where added sugar is coming in.

PREPPING YOURSELF

If you're up for doing some light cooking on weeknights, spend some time over the weekend selecting a couple of no-nonsense recipes for the week, then make sure you have the right ingredients on hand. Meals at home become a whole lot easier to make when you invest your energy in light meal prep—for instance, having certain key elements ready to go, such as roasted sweet potatoes, spiralized zucchini, riced cauliflower, store-bought organic rotisserie chicken, hard-boiled eggs, sliced raw veggies, and some dips. This way, you can assemble different dishes or whip up meals on the spot by tweaking the flavor profile to suit what you're craving (such as throwing together zoodles, dairy-free pesto, and rotisserie chicken, or cauliflower rice, sesame oil, kimchi, and veggies, with an egg on top).

That's what one of my clients, Jenna, learned to do. A working mom who had a particularly tough time with planning and preparing dinner, Jenna loved cooking but felt overwhelmed by the sheer number of recipes she had pinned and screen-shot on her phone. By the time she got home from work and decided on one, a take-out delivery order was often already en route. She had previously been in the habit of going to the farmers' market every Sunday, but she didn't always use the produce she bought, so she gradually stopped going altogether because she felt guilty about wasting food. As a result, there were never any fresh veggies on hand that she could use to concoct a healthy dinner.

In Jenna's case, the solution was fairly straightforward: creating structure and offering herself a hefty dose of self-compassion. To kick the habit of subjecting herself to the (self-imposed) pressure of creating new dishes every week, we sat down and made a list of her favorite dishes to prepare and put them on a rotation schedule. The deal was that she could experiment once a week if she felt inspired, but it wasn't something she *had* to do in order to feel successful. With this approach, she'd know what she was cooking ahead of time, so she could Instacart the ingredients while she was still at work. For Jenna, the second part of the challenge was to ditch the guilt about potentially wasting food. We can all agree that wasting food is something we'd rather not do it—but, hey, sometimes it happens. In Jenna's case, the guilt about potentially wasting food was preventing her from stocking up on fresh produce. By letting go of that guilt, she was able to focus her attention on setting herself up to have the healthy ingredients she needed on hand for the week.

To make cooking at home efficient, think about how to organize your kitchen so you can access those healthy ingredients quickly. Also, consider how you can limit mindless nibbling while you're cooking: For example, keep tempting but not-so-healthy foods off your countertops and in opaque containers so they're harder to get to and less enticing; instead, keep good-for-you snacks (like crudités and roasted veggies) at eye level in your fridge. Remember the crudités trick from Chapter 4? It really, seriously works, but only if the veggies are already washed and cut.

Simply put: When you're hungry for a snack, you're not going to want to do any legwork (as in rinsing and slicing); in those moments, it's much easier to choose something in your pantry, fridge, or freezer that doesn't involve any effort. So get in the routine of having crudités available: As soon as you get back from the market (or have your groceries delivered), wash and cut your veggies and place them front and center in your fridge. After a while, you'll start to notice that it takes less and less effort to prep them, place them, and reach for them. Hey, you might even start to look forward to the ritual. *Just saying.*

EATING GROUND = SACRED GROUND

When I was an undergrad, I was an especially bad sleeper; mostly, I had a hard time falling asleep. In addition to learning good sleep hygiene, one of the best pieces of advice I got was to avoid difficult convos in bed. The same principle goes for the dining table: If you want to develop and maintain healthy-eating habits, avoid having stressful chats (about what's missing from your sex life, the state of your finances, and other cortisol-igniting subjects) while you're eating. Make an effort to relax before you eat, and then focus on enjoying your food.

Also, if your dining table is where you usually place your mail and your laptop, or you can't actually see the kitchen counters, you'd be wise to do some rearranging. Clutter like this can create a chaotic eating environment that encourages overeating. In a study published in the February 2016 issue of *Environment and Behavior*, researchers found that women consumed *twice* as many cookies in a messy kitchen—with newspapers on the table and dirty dishes, pots, and pans in the sink—than in an organized one. It's as if they were internalizing the kitchen chaos.

When You're at Work

Perpetually winging it at lunchtime can make it especially hard to stick with your get-healthy goals; in fact, you could be inadvertently undermining some of the healthy strides you've been making. I hear a version of this scenario a lot: Someone wants to eat healthier lunches at work, but he or she doesn't think about *where* to get healthy options that will be truly enjoyable to eat. As a result, the person often ends up at a place with not-so-great options and is forced to settle on something unsatisfying. Worse, he or she comes to associate eating healthfully with feeling frustrated or disappointed. If you want to eat more healthfully at work, think about where you'll get your meal: Are there places nearby with options you'll actually enjoy? Will you bring leftovers from home? Is there a fridge at work where you can store basics like veggies and dip?

When You're on the Go

Keep healthy snacks—such as prepackaged roasted nuts, nori strips, sweet potato chips, and toasted coconut flakes—in your car, bag, and desk so you never go famished. Other great homemade favorites include energy bites (see page 165), spicy kale chips, plantain chips, and clean trail mix combos like wasabi peas, roasted nuts, and refined-sugar-free dark chocolate chunks. Having satisfying nibbles on hand is especially helpful for days when you know you won't have time to eat at normal times. I'm not saying you should make a habit out of snacking on trail mix for lunch, but sometimes you just don't have time to eat until late afternoon, and during those times, grab-and-go items like these come in particularly handy.

STRATEGIC SHORTCUTS

I work with lots of different types of busy folks, and in a parallel universe free of obligations, many of them would love to make complex dinners on the regular. But that's just not real life right now. Hearing variations of their cooking-guilt conundrums inspired me to adopt a somewhat scrappy approach to dinner that involves minimal effort when time is scarce because, let's be real: Sometimes you just crave something that feels homemade. Here are three great strategies for doing this:

Doctoring Up Premade Foods

I'm all about sprucing up high-quality grocery-store items (mostly pre-prepared) and making them feel special and at least a *little* fussed-over. I'm talking about stuff like storebought organic rotisserie chicken, cooked quinoa, and riced cauliflower, which you can either sauté quickly with aromatics like shallots, onions, and garlic, use for stir-fries and soups, *or* use meal-assembly style for stuff like bowls, salads, and lettuce-wrapped tacos. Better yet, throw a little rosemary and thyme, crispy sage, dairy-free pesto, tahini, or curry powder on there, and *boom*—now we're talking! You've made it your own.

Batch-Ordering from Restaurants

You've probably heard of batch cooking, but what about batch ordering? If you're out to dinner, or ordering in, peek at the menu to see if there's anything that may come in handy later on. In addition to double ordering for leftover lunch the next day, check to see if there are any sides with repurpose potential. For example, if there's a simple baked sweet potato on a menu and I've got a particularly busy week ahead of me, I'll often order a couple to use throughout the week, cubed in salads and Buddha bowls, and blended in soups, smoothies, dips, and chia seed pudding. Extra roasted veggies left over after a dinner out? Grab them for stuff like stir-fries and stews that you make at home.

Making Multitasking Ingredients

If you're taking the time to cook something at home, do yourself a favor and focus on foods with real multitasking utility for the week. Take salmon, for instance, which can be used in anything from cauliflower "fried" rice to salmon tacos, salads, and collard wraps to omelets. The same thing goes for clean sauces and dips like pesto, turmeric tahini, and green goddess dressing, which, much like a little black dress, can pretty much go with anything. For instance, if you opt to make homemade dairy-free pesto, you can use it to make scrambled eggs a little more special, or put it on kelp noodles, or drizzle on sliced tomatoes and avocado for a simple snack. As you'll discover in Chapter 7, you may even start thinking of certain foods as staple wardrobe pieces that you can mix and match and enjoy often.

REVAMPING YOUR FOOD RITUALS

We all have automatic noshing tendencies that are (knowingly or not) part of our regularly scheduled lives. The trouble is, certain food-centric scenarios—girls' night in, watching a movie, or scrolling through Instagram late at night—can trigger overeating by creating a case of classical conditioning (like Pavlov and his dogs). If you're used to having nachos and margaritas at your monthly book club meeting with your besties, you might be engaging in hand-to-mouth activity without much thought. But you can upgrade these tendencies by arming yourself with better choices.

Don't panic: This doesn't mean you have to replace nachos with carrot sticks—but you can supplement with healthier options that will still pack serious flavor. The first step is to identify recurring situations where overeating is practically a reflex, then upgrade or vary your snack options. For example:

During ladies' night: Instead of making starchy fare the food staple for the evening, switch things up now and then with fresh-cut veggies and guac, homemade kale or beet chips, cauliflower popcorn, or even a more complex carb like sweet potato fries with tahini.

At the movies: I would *never* recommend bringing apple slices or a baggie of celery to the movies when you really want candy (what a joke!)—but you *can* bring a better-for-you substitute like dark chocolate and hazelnuts. This way, you can enjoy a tasty treat but without all the extra sugar and other unnecessary stuff that's in movie theatre candy these days.

During dinner prep or your kids' mealtime: Do you tend to be so ravenous by the late afternoon that you end up snacking while you cook or picking from your kids' plates during an early dinner—and basically consume the equivalent of a small meal before the main event? Well, here's a better approach:

(continued on next page)

Munch from a plate of raw veggies while you cook or keep the kids company—and consider this your amuse-bouche.

While scrolling through your phone late at night: First, question whether you're actually hungry. If you are, have a delish but not sugar-laden pre-bedtime snack (such as coconut milk hot chocolate with a handful of roasted cashews). If you're not, but you're fixated on getting some oral satisfaction anyway, treat yourself to a cup of warm nut milk with cinnamon or vanilla extract or tea sans caffeine.

STEALTH TIP

If you're a perpetual late-night snacker, flossing and brushing your teeth right after your meal can be a deterrent to further munching. The reason: Having to re-floss and re-brush your pearly whites is enough of an inconvenience to act as a roadblock for noshing on stuff that's not really worth it to you.

When I'm working with clients, the themes of structure and planning always take center stage. These organizing principles scale back the need for constant willpower and decision-making, and start to streamline healthy behaviors. Even better, when we provide ourselves with enough structure (like having predetermined recipes and a well-stocked kitchen), it actually helps us to be *more* flexible, because we don't have to reinvent the wheel, meal after meal. Instead of squeezing out every last ounce of willpower each night as you decide whether to eat something healthy (or not), you're better off frontloading some time and energy, making sure you have the components of healthy, enjoyable meals on hand; this way, you'll be ready to go for the next couple of days. As with anything else, the more often you do something, the more automated the behavior becomes, and when you automate (in a good way) some of your eating decisions, less effort is required to make consciously healthy food choices on the regular. *And why not make life easier?*

Just as it's unrealistic to expect your romantic relationship to be flawless 365 days a year, it's unfair to expect yourself to make perfectly thoughtful food decisions, meal after meal, day after day. Like any muscle, willpower can be fatigued with overuse, but it can also be conserved and bolstered, in this case by sidestepping temptations and precommitting to healthy choices ahead of time. By taking the pressure-easing steps in this chapter, you'll be setting yourself up to stay true to your intentions and have a less conflicted, more harmonious relationship with food. *And who doesn't want that?* Once you get your hormones working in your favor, as you'll learn to do in the next chapter, this feel-good goal will be that much easier to achieve.

PART TWO

YOUR DELICIOUSLY DOABLE FOOD INTERVENTION

6

Get Your Hormones Working for You with the Food Therapist Plan

Many of our most basic desires are driven by hormonal activity—whether we're craving cake, espresso, a quickie, or deep sleep. But when it comes to relationships, hormones can work for *or* against us. When they're working for us, there's nothing quite like it...we're talking butterflies, and that can't-keep-your-hands-to-yourself lust. Maybe you've heard about the "bonding" hormone: oxytocin, which fosters trust and attachment in relationships, including between lovers, and also between mothers and their newborn babes. Hugging, snuggling, spooning, and other forms of physical affection can all stimulate an oxytocin rush, triggering that blissed-out feeling. In happy times, the effects feel pretty incredible.

At the same time, if you've ever short-fused on your significant other for something relatively harmless—when you're overtired, overworked, or underfed—then you know that hormones can also make us act out in *less-than-ideal* ways. In fact, oxytocin can also trigger feelings of jealousy, envy, and fury when things aren't going so hot. Let's face it: Whenever negative emotions are running particularly high, there's a good chance that hormones like cortisol are worked up, too. It's during those times—discovering your S.O. text-flirted with another gal, or when you're feeling volatile due to lack of sleep, stress, or in adequate sustenance—that fiery passion often overrides rationality, and we tend to say and do things we don't actually mean. As you may have guessed or can recall from personal experience, hormonally fueled scenarios like these often encourage us to eat things we don't intend to, as well.

A little background: Hormones are chemical messengers that regulate everything from our energy levels, appetite, fat storage, and metabolism to our stress levels and sex drive. We all have natural sensors in our brains, fat cells, and other organs that keep tabs on hormone levels in our bloodstream, kind of like extra-alert watchdogs. These internal monitors are really good at picking up on when something in the body is out of balance—for instance, when there's suddenly an excess of sugar in the bloodstream after eating Swedish Fish at the movies. That's when specialized sensors prompt the pancreas to release the hormone insulin in order to escort the considerable sugar overflow to its proper place (namely, out of the bloodstream). This system of checks and balances is in perpetual motion, because the body is *constantly* trying to achieve a harmonious equilibrium. There's good reason for that, because the human body works *really* well when it's in a balanced state. During those even-keeled times, our hormones are reliable gauges that tell us when we're low on fuel and need to eat, and when to put down our forks. But when the system is out of balance... not so much. When our hormones are off-kilter, our fat storage amps up, our stress signals spike, our metabolism slows, and our instinct to lunge for sugar kicks in, and yet our fullness signals don't quite register. Not to be too dramatic, but it's kind of like a *Homeland* plotline playing out in our bodies on continuous loop. I promise we can solve this, but first let's take a closer look at some of the major hormones at play in regulating hunger, fullness, and body weight.

Insulin: When it comes to hormones that affect our weight, insulin is a *biggie*, and that's because it decides whether the food we eat is stored as quick fuel for energy or as body fat. Think of insulin as the ultra-organized and efficient Virgo neat freak whose job is to keep blood sugar in check. To continue with the movie-noshing example: When you have some Swedish Fish occasionally, insulin responds to the influx of sugar in the bloodstream and stores it away kind of like a light jacket...something you don't exactly need right now, but also something you'll want to keep in an accessible place like a hallway closet, so you can grab it quickly should you need it. In your body, the form of sugar that's stored like a light jacket is called glycogen, which is housed in the liver and the muscles and is easily broken down for fuel. When your diet is balanced and your hormones are in sync, insulin generally stores some sugar as glycogen in the liver, a bunch in the muscles, and little to none in fat cells.

The issue is that there's only a finite amount of storage space available to stash sugar this way. If we end up eating too much sugar and carbs consistently (for instance, Swedish Fish every day), insulin has to work overtime and it morphs into a pretty efficient fat-storing hormone to keep up. It's as if you lived in a studio apartment and bought ten new pairs of shoes every day: Even if you were giving a couple of pairs away on a daily basis, eventually you'd run out of space in your more easily accessible storage areas. Shoes would start piling up, and you'd have to switch gears and start warehousing the surplus in a bigger, more long-term facility (like the creepy one in the basement of my building). In the body, that long-term storage facility is inside our fat cells, which are extra good at expanding to accommodate the glucose overflow; the trouble is, it's more difficult to convince our fat cells to shrink and unload the excess, Marie Kondo style. Anyone who has ever had to deal with a remote storage facility *or* excess fat storage knows the struggle is real. Aside from amping up fat accrual, consistent insulin surges prompt other hormones to autocorrect in a not-so-great way. Enter cortisol...

Cortisol: Cortisol is kind of like the 911 hormone that's released into the bloodstream when our bodies perceive a legit threat on deck. But as I mentioned, our hormonal sensors are supervigilant, and they're known to sound the cortisol alarm for just about anything, from stress to things the body mislabels as dangerous, like intense workouts, missing lunch, and food sensitivities. When high insulin levels aren't in the picture, the presence of cortisol isn't a big deal; in fact, we need a certain amount of cortisol just to get out of bed in the morning. But when elevated cortisol is paired with elevated insulin levels, it's basically like two fat-storage-promoting villains joining forces. Besides making us crave sugar, cortisol further cranks up insulin levels and makes insulin *even more* efficient at storing fat. In doing so, it also mucks with the hormones that control our appetite (namely, leptin and ghrelin), making us feel perpetually hungry.

Leptin: When we eat, the hormone leptin is released by the fat cells and travels to the brain to announce that we've had enough. An internal fullness gauge that keeps us from overeating—*amazing*. The problem is that excess insulin and cortisol can dull leptin's signal, so the brain doesn't actually receive the message that we're full, and we continue eating. *Anyone relate?* The same thing happens when we don't get adequate shut-eye. Leptin levels surge during deep, restorative sleep, which is why skimping on zzz's is so often correlated with a case of the munchies and weight gain. Meanwhile, amplified cortisol and insulin levels and too little sleep also happen to crank up ghrelin, a hormone that revs up appetite. It helps to think of the two hormones—leptin and ghrelin—as forming a powerful checks-and-balances system: one handles appetite, the other handles satiety. We want them both to work effectively, naturally, and harmoniously—and it's up to us to create an environment inside our bodies that encourages this to go down. When it does, relying on our body's hunger and fullness cues gets easier, and our relationship with food and our bodies isn't quite as complicated.

To drive this point home, let's look at the flip side for a moment: Let's say you want to gain a lot of body fat (*I know, I get it*—it's an unlikely scenario, but just go with it): Your best bet would be to keep insulin levels high throughout the day, which would throw your leptin and ghrelin levels out of whack. An easy way to do this would be to eat lots of foods that are straight-up sugar *or* perpetually overdo it on carbs that are broken down into sugar fairly rapidly—fiber-lacking foods like processed cereal, white pasta, white bread, and white rice, excess fruit, and sugary beverages (yes, including fresh-pressed organic ones). When we eat these foods, blood sugar levels sky-rocket, and since it's up to insulin to deal with keeping excess sugar out of the bloodstream, it stores the spillover as efficiently as possible, often as body fat. *Not the goal here!* That's why I'm all about preventing this scenario by avoiding dramatic blood sugar surges and keeping these hormones in check.

As you may be gleaning, these powerful weight-balance hormones are pretty interconnected. When the equilibrium isn't quite right, the whole system is thrown off course, increasing your chances of packing on unwanted pounds, not to mention keeping your body's metabolic engine stuck in neutral or reverse. But the really good news is that the opposite is also true: When you reset insulin levels, the hormones that regulate your metabolism and your appetite will normalize, too. *Seriously, though, how great is that?*

So the question is: How do you reboot insulin? The answer: Know your carbs. Pick your carbohydrates prudently, focusing on high-quality, slow-burn sources (ones that trigger a gradual, steady release of insulin versus a rapid spike), keep your portions in check, and space them out over time; also, pair these smart carbs with healthy fats, fiber, and high-quality protein, which will help buffer the insulin surge. Bottom line: If you keep your blood sugar in check consistently, you'll improve your insulin, leptin, and ghrelin levels—and your body will start working *for* you rather than against you.

THE FOOD THERAPIST PLAN

The Food Therapist Plan that follows is all about encouraging your hormones to work in service of your get-healthy goals for a change—to tame constant cravings and help you feel your best. This modified Paleo approach, which can be tweaked for most eating styles except vegan, helps you lose weight or maintain the healthy weight you want without feeling deprived or constantly hungry (an anomaly, I know). The plan has two phases: Phase I is designed specifically to reset your hormones; Phase II maintains that reset and broadens your carb options, so you can apply it sustainably in real life.

Put another way: Phase I is really a reboot that helps your

body get back to its natural harmonious, balanced state. It's about eating in a way that will make your body as friendly an environment as possible so your hormones can start working as they're meant to. During Phase I, which lasts three weeks because that's roughly how long it takes for your hormones to make the adjustment, you'll ditch gluten, grains, white potatoes, corn, legumes, refined sugar, artificial sugar, lactose, soy, and alcohol. But I assure you: You won't be going hungry. Since you'll be boosting your healthy fat intake from flavorful, filling foods like rich sauces and creamy dips, avocados and nuts, you'll be plenty satisfied while you're fine-tuning your insulin and hunger hormones and keeping inflammation at bay.

If you're wondering why gluten, grains, corn, legumes, soy, and dairy foods get the boot in Phase I, here's the scoop: Many grains (especially wheat) and legumes (especially soybeans and peanuts) contain lectins, proteins that can lead to sneaky, harmful inflammation in the body. While most foods contain some lectins, there are a handful of foods— including grains, legumes, and dairy products from grain-fed animals—that contain *a lot* of them.* We have a rough time digesting lectins because they are clingy in our digestive tracts and are prone to attaching to our intestinal walls. This is a problem because the intestinal lining works kind of like the bouncer at a nightclub door, deciding what's allowed to

---

* FYI: Nightshades (white potatoes, tomatoes, eggplants, peppers, and goji berries) are also abundant in lectins but tend to be less problematic, so I've left them in to keep this plan sustainable.

enter and pass into the bloodstream and what's not. Many different characters—including essential nutrients, bacteria and viruses, and inflammatory proteins like lectins—are vying for admission, and in order for the gatekeeper to be tough and discerning, the gut lining needs to be healthy.

When the lining of the gut is healthy, the structure is so tightly woven that it's only permeable by small molecules—and that's a good thing. When it's not so healthy or when it's irritated, the intestinal lining can become more porous, allowing things to seep into the bloodstream that don't belong there—like undigested food particles and lectins. When this happens, the body attacks these particles as if they were pathogens (aka germs that make us sick), which can trigger inflammation inside us. If this happens repeatedly over time, you're looking at the possibility of food allergies and sensitivities, and in some cases impaired insulin sensitivity and leptin production. This is when you might experience the vague and not-so-flirty symptoms of bloating, cramps, fatigue, constant hunger and sugar cravings, weight gain, and inflammatory skin conditions like eczema and rosacea. Everyone is different, but gluten-containing grains and cow's milk dairy products are some of the more common offenders.

Take a breath! This doesn't mean you can't ever have another grain or bean or spoonful of yogurt again. But for Phase I of the plan, I recommend temporarily ditching these foods in order to give your body a chance to relax, regroup, and rebalance itself internally. That said, if you are a vegetarian who doesn't eat fish, I recommend keeping dried beans and legumes—ideally, soaked before cooking, because these versions have lower lectin concentrations—in your diet in Phase I in order to ensure that you're getting enough protein. After three weeks, you'll move into Phase II and you can add some of these foods back in to your meals.

In Phase II, which lasts for one week, you can add back beans and legumes (again, ideally soaked and boiled), gluten-free grains (like brown rice and whole oats), high-quality, high-fat dairy products, corn, peanuts, and one glass of alcohol per day if you fancy it. It's best to reintroduce these foods slowly (meaning, not all at one meal) so you'll have a better chance of pinpointing how you're reacting to each one. For the record, I don't recommend consuming processed soy products (like tofu, tempeh, soy milk, soy-based protein powder, and "fake" meats) on a regular basis: Soy contains plant-based compounds called isoflavones that are structurally similar to estrogen, which means they can disrupt the body's natural hormonal balance. This isn't a big deal when you consume moderate amounts of unprocessed organic soybeans like edamame, which are an incredible source of protein for vegetarians. But it's easy to overdo it with processed soy foods, which aren't as nutritious anyway. The goal for Phase II is to continue resetting your hormones but also to figure out what works for you. You may find that, like me, you feel better without grains and dairy altogether, but can tolerate some legumes quite well, especially the sprouted and fermented varieties, like dosa. On the other hand, it's totally possible that you'll feel fine incorporating all of the above.

As you're bringing previously shelved foods back to your plate, pay attention to how you feel and adjust your approach accordingly. If having yogurt or a whole-grain pasta leaves you feeling foggy, sluggish, or bloated, or your GI tract is sending distress signals, it's up to you to choose whether (or when) it's worth it to you to eat those foods.

With this in mind, after the Phase II week is up, you're welcome to incorporate a broader range of other carbs in moderation. Will your body feel and function as well if you replace all your smart carb servings with bagels and alcohol? Absolutely not. But at the same time, it's important for me to show you how things like bagels and alcohol can fit into your diet so that you don't feel like you have to make an all-or-nothing choice. The idea is to mix and match carbs so that this plan works for you in a flexible, sustainable way. It's kind of like having a not-so-rigid parenting style— giving your kids enough freedom and flexibility so they're less inclined to straight-up revolt.

Once you get the hang of divvying up your carb servings, you'll be able to choose delicious, healthy foods throughout the day that are in line with your long-term goals without overthinking it. One of the main reasons the Food Therapist Plan is so effective is that when you improve your carb game (choosing high-quality ones, spacing them out, and not going overboard), your insulin levels don't end up in overdrive. This means you're encouraging your body to burn excess fat instead of storing it; moreover, insulin doesn't have a chance to mess with your leptin and ghrelin levels. *Now we're talking.*

THE FOOD THERAPIST PLAN CHEAT SHEET

If your head is spinning from all this info, here's a simple guide to help you navigate what to eat (and ditch) in both phases.

Phase I (3 weeks)

Foods to savor	Foods to avoid
Veggies: All except corn and white potatoes	***Veggies:*** Corn, white potatoes
Alternative dairy products: Hemp milk, coconut milk, nut milk, ghee	***Dairy:*** Milk, butter, whey protein, yogurt, cheese
Grains: Quinoa	***Grains:*** All except quinoa
Oils: MCT, coconut, olive, avocado, flax, sesame, almond, walnut, hazelnut, and pumpkin seed oils	***Oils:*** Margarine, shortening; corn, soy, sunflower, safflower, and canola oils
Beverages: Filtered/sparkling/ mineral water, unsweetened tea, high-quality unsweetened coffee (feel free to add ghee, MCT oil, or coconut oil)	***Beverages:*** Alcohol, fruit juice, sweetened or artificially sweetened beverages, rice milk, soy milk
	Vegetable proteins: Beans and legumes, hummus, processed soybean products (soy milk, soy sauce, tofu, tempeh, seitan)
Animal proteins: Wild fish, oil-packed anchovies, organic or pasture-raised eggs, free-range poultry, and grass-fed meats	***Animal proteins:*** Processed meats
Nuts and seeds: All except peanuts and sweetened nut and seed butters	***Nuts and seeds:*** Peanuts, peanut butter, and sweetened nut and seed butters
Sweeteners: Coconut nectar/sugar, maple syrup, raw honey, and stevia (max 1 Tbsp. per day)	***Sweeteners:*** Agave, processed and refined sugar, artificial sweeteners

Condiments: Apple cider vinegar, white wine vinegar, balsamic vinegar, brown rice vinegar, Champagne vinegar, coconut aminos, tahini, gluten-free fish sauce, Dijon mustard, sauerkraut, kimchi, unsweetened mayo, dairy-free pesto, hot sauce, Karam's Garlic Sauce (page 85), Majestic Garlic Spread (page 85)	**Condiments:** Any condiment containing gluten or soy (like soy sauce), or any of the above sweeteners or ingredients
Fruit: All fruits except sweetened, canned, and dried	**Fruit:** Sweetened, canned, and dried fruits like raisins, dried mango, dried apricots, and dried cranberries

Phase II (1 week)

Foods to savor	Foods to avoid
Veggies: All except white potatoes	**Veggies:** White potatoes
Dairy: High-quality, full-fat dairy like kefir, whole milk, Greek yogurt, cream, and cheese	**Dairy:** Reduced- and low-fat dairy products, yogurt with added refined sugar or artificial sweeteners
Alternative dairy products: Hemp milk, coconut milk, nut milk, ghee	
Grains: Gluten-free whole grains like quinoa, brown rice, whole oats, amaranth, buckwheat, millet, sorghum, and teff	**Grains:** Glutinous grains like wheat, bulgur, farro, spelt, kamut, barley, and rye; refined grains like white rice
Oils: MCT, coconut, olive, avocado, flax, sesame, almond, walnut, hazelnut, and pumpkin seed oils	**Oils:** Margarine, shortening; corn, soy, sunflower, safflower, and canola oils
Beverages: Filtered/sparkling/mineral water, unsweetened tea, high-quality unsweetened coffee (feel free to add ghee, MCT oil, or coconut oil to make it Bulletproof style)	**Beverages:** Fruit juice, sweetened or artificially sweetened beverages, soy milk

(continued on next page)

Foods to savor	Foods to avoid
Alcohol: Gluten-free beer, sake, dry wine and Champagne, rum, tequila, potato vodka (1 glass max per day)	**Alcohol:** Gluten-containing and sweetened
Vegetable proteins: Legumes and beans like peanuts, chickpeas, black-eyed peas, lentils, red beans, black beans, kidney beans, white beans, and hummus	**Vegetable proteins:** Processed soybean products (soy milk, soy sauce, tofu, tempeh, seitan)
Animal proteins: Wild fish, oil-packed anchovies, organic or pasture-raised eggs, free-range poultry, and grass-fed meats	**Animal proteins:** Processed meats
Nuts and seeds: All except sweetened nut and seed butters	**Nuts and seeds:** Sweetened nut and seed butters
Sweeteners: Coconut nectar/sugar, maple syrup, raw honey, and stevia (max 1 Tbsp. per day)	**Sweeteners:** Agave, processed and refined sugar, artificial sweeteners
Condiments: Apple cider vinegar, white wine vinegar, balsamic vinegar, brown rice vinegar, Champagne vinegar, coconut aminos, tahini, gluten-free fish sauce, Dijon mustard, sauerkraut, kimchi, unsweetened mayo, dairy-free pesto, hot sauce, Karam's Garlic Sauce (page 85), Majestic Garlic Spread (page 85)	**Condiments:** Any condiment containing gluten or soy (like soy sauce), or any of the above sweeteners or ingredients
Fruit: All fruits except sweetened, canned, and dried	**Fruit:** Sweetened, canned, and dried fruits

Note: You'll still want to avoid soy-based foods, gluten-containing foods, refined sugar, refined grains, white potatoes, and processed foods.

What About Calories?

You've probably heard the debate about whether all calories are created equal. This plan focuses on carbs, *not* calories, and here's why: In the lab, a calorie *is*, in fact, a calorie, meaning that 500 calories from OJ (carbs) or olive oil (fat) will each release the same amount of energy when torched on the trusty Bunsen burner (that's how scientists measure calories, btw). But in the body that equation doesn't compute because of the way foods behave once they're inside us. Different foods have varying effects on the hormones that control our cravings, hunger, satiety, metabolism, blood sugar, and fat storage. For instance, because the body can't actually break down all the fiber contained in carbs like sweet potatoes (as opposed to a less fibrous source like white rice), the carbs in a fiber-rich food don't cause as substantial a spike in blood sugar and insulin.

When it comes to how foods impact insulin (and therefore fat storage) the most, there's a hierarchy: Fiber-lacking refined carbs that are broken down quickly have the most dramatic impact on insulin; protein has a minimal effect; and dietary fat has no effect at all. That's why in putting together a balanced diet I recommend using this hierarchy to inform your plate, leading with non-starchy veggies (like leafy greens, zoodles, and cauliflower rice) topped with a generous helping of delicious high-quality fat (such as olive oil, ghee, avocado, and the rich sauces you'll find in the next chapter); then you can add high-quality protein (4 to 6 ounces of cooked free-range organic chicken, turkey, grass-fed lamb, wild salmon, or 2 eggs) in a supporting role, and fiber-rich complex carbs like sweet potatoes and quinoa as key guest stars.

In short, monitoring calories doesn't matter all that much, but managing hormones, particularly insulin, really does. Eating the right kinds of fat while avoiding pro-inflammatory, hormone-disrupting trans fats and limiting highly processed oils (like corn, soy, sunflower, safflower, and canola) can really help the cause because they don't affect insulin, but they do help keep us full and make everything tastier. Until fairly recently, health experts pushed calorie-restricted, low-fat diets for weight loss. The main problem with these diets—aside from being absolutely dreadful—is that they simply don't work: Eating ample amounts of high-quality fat is the key to losing (and/or maintaining a healthy) weight and enjoying the process; plus, dietary fat speeds up your metabolism, mediates insulin surges, and helps keep cravings at bay. Many of the same effects are true of protein. As for carbs, yes, you do need them, but it's a delicate balance: Eating too few carbs will make you feel tired and cranky and can actually crank up cortisol production; on the other hand, having too many carbs, especially from concentrated sugar and processed starches, leads to dramatic insulin surges, which amps up fat storage and throws off the other key hormones. So you'll want to find your sweet spot, which this plan will help you master.

We all vary in how we respond to carbs, but I've found that most women do best when they hover in the 60-to-90-gram range, broken down into four to six servings (of roughly 15 grams each) throughout the day. Generally speaking, six servings puts you in the sweet spot for weight maintenance, while four to five servings puts you in the zone for weight loss. Of course, if you're exercising intensely (such as training for a serious athletic event) or if you're pregnant or nursing, you'll need to add more servings of carbs. Keep in mind that this is real life, so think of a carb serving as somewhere in the 13-to-22-gram range.

The Carb Swap Meet

I became a believer in this plan when I was completing my dietetic residency at Mount Sinai Medical Center in Manhattan. In the hospital, I had the opportunity to teach people who were newly diagnosed with type 1 diabetes how to keep track of and space out their carbs in order to figure out how much insulin they'd need to administer after eating. Those with type 1 diabetes don't make enough insulin naturally, so they have to take it as medicine after consuming carb-containing meals to usher sugar out of their bloodstream (otherwise, it would start piling up). In their case, minding carb servings isn't just healthy—it's *crucial*. Of course, finding out you have any chronic illness really sucks, but type 1 diabetes can feel especially burdensome because, as you can imagine, it requires constant planning, thought, and maintenance; plus, for many people, the prospect of keeping track of and limiting carbs indefinitely can feel like a complete and total punishment.

So here's what I'd tell them: *I know this is overwhelming, but if it makes you feel even an ounce better, just about everyone would be a whole lot healthier and better off divvying up carb servings this way; it's just that unfortunately the stakes of not eating this way are higher for you.* To be honest, I'm not sure if that provided any solace, but as I worked with more patients and did my own research, I became more convinced than ever of the universal advantages of this approach. So when I started my private practice, I began using my own take on the carb-exchange method with every client because it's really *that* healthy and user-friendly. Another perk: It gets rid of the "what's a portion" guessing game, which tends to trip so many of us up.

If you get used to thinking of carbs in terms of 15-gram servings, you can figure out how they fit into your daily four-, five-, or six-serving budget. It's really about deciding where you want to "spend" your carb servings. Plus, you'll be able to look at virtually any food label and figure out how many carb servings are in a portion (based on the 15-gram guideline). What follows is a look at what 15 grams of carbs looks like in terms of actual food. The list gives you ideas for how to divvy up carbs throughout the day, in both Phase I and Phase II of the plan.

I find that most clients feel their best on a pseudo 80/20 Paleo breakdown, eating a diet that's mostly light on gluten, grains, dairy, and refined sugar, but not so rigid that they are *forbidden* from indulging in those things when it feels right to them. So don't be afraid to play around with carb-serving combos, because that flexibility is part of what makes this plan work for so many people: You could have two carb servings in the morning (a Super-Simple Smoothie on page 159 or a gluten-free English muffin smothered with nut butter or ghee), one at lunch (chickpeas on a well-dressed big salad with protein), a low-carb dinner (cauliflower tortilla fish tacos with spicy slaw and guac), and one for dark chocolate and a glass of dry red vino after dinner. Or, you could borrow the strategy boss lady Jenna Lyons, former president and creative director of J. Crew, calls her "lunch uniform": Eating a similar (low-carb) lunch every day, which means you'd save your carb flexibility for breakfast, dinner, and snacks. The upside is that this approach can help reduce decision fatigue. The downside is that it can be monotonous (but you can spice it up with the strategies in Chapter 8). So it's your call whether you try it out.

Carb Price Tags

Imagine that you have a smart-carb spending allowance, rather than unlimited funds: Keeping track of your carb price tags will help you manage and balance your budget. Over time, it will support the ultimate goal: Being able to guesstimate servings so you're not bogged down with the details and can focus on tuning in to yourself and enjoying your food. But to get there, you'll want to get familiar with what a carb serving actually looks like. So let's cut to the chase. What follows is a list of carb-containing foods that can be eaten in Phase I, Phase II, or both:

Starchy Veggies (both phases)

Beets: 1 cup
Jicama: 1½ cups
Peas: ¾ cup

Pumpkin (no sugar added): 1 cup
Sweet potato and taro root chips: 1 ounce
Winter squash (acorn, butternut): 1 cup
Yam and sweet potato: ½ medium or ½ cup chunks

Grains and Beans (Phase II)

Brown rice: ⅓ cup cooked
Quinoa: ⅓ cup cooked (Phase I friendly, because it's technically
    a seed)
Beans and lentils: ½ cup cooked
Edamame: ¾ cup
Hummus: ⅓ cup
Oatmeal (cooked old-fashioned oats, unsweetened): ½ cup
Bagel: ¼ typical bagel (yep, a typical bagel contains 4 carb servings)
Corn: ½ cup kernels or 6-inch cob
English muffin: ½
Most sliced breads: 1 slice
Popcorn: 3 cups (not bad)
Standard rice cakes: 2
Pasta: ⅓ cup cooked
Rice milk, unsweetened: 6 ounces
Tortilla (6-inch): 1
Siete Foods Grain Free Tortilla Chips: 9 (see Pantry Essentials)

Fruits (both phases)

Apple: 1 small
Apricots (fresh): 4 small
Banana: ½ large or 1 baby

Blackberries: ¾ cup

Blueberries: ¾ cup

Cantaloupe: 1 cup cubes

Cherries: ½ cup

Dates: 1 medjool or 3 small deglet noor

Grapefruit: ½ medium

Grapes: 1 cup

Honeydew: 1 cup cubes

Kiwi: 2 small

Mango: ½ small or ½ cup chunks

Mulberries: 1 cup

Nectarine: 1 medium

Orange: 1 small

Papaya: 1 cup cubes

Peach: 1 large

Pear: 1 small

Pineapple: ¾ cup cubes

Plum: 2 small

Pomegranate: ½ cup seeds

Raspberries: 1 cup

Strawberries: 1¼ cups

Tangerine: 2 small

Watermelon: 1¼ cups cubes

Miscellaneous

Unsweetened full-fat coconut milk: 1 cup (Phase I friendly)

Coconut sugar, maple syrup, raw honey, blackstrap molasses:
    1 tablespoon (Phase I friendly, up to 1 tablespoon per day)

Jelly and jam: 1 tablespoon (Phase II only)

All fruit juice: ⅓ cup (Phase II only; keep this in mind next time
   you're ordering a Mimosa or other juicy cocktail)

Free Foods (go wild: you can have as much as you like of these)

All green veggies (including broccoli), leafy greens
Brussels sprouts
Cabbage
Carrots
Cauliflower
Cucumber
Eggplant
Garlic
Ginger
Green beans
Herbs
Lime and lemon juice/zest
Mushrooms
Onions
Peppers
Pepperoncini (my personal fave)
Radishes
Sauerkraut
Seaweed (kelp, wakame, etc.)
Snap peas
Spices
Sprouts (all kinds)
Squash (summer, zucchini)

Tomatoes

Unsweetened veggie juice

Water chestnuts

THE BOOZE FACTOR

It's true that alcohol contains carbs, but not all types carry a hefty carb price tag. If you plan on incorporating adult beverages during Phase II and beyond, keep in mind that gluten-free spirits like tequila and vodka and dry Champagnes and wines are your best bets. Don't drive yourself crazy trying to crunch the numbers (that's a major buzzkill, to say the least). But do take a minute to familiarize yourself with the general breakdown by perusing this cheat sheet on the average carb price tags of various forms of alcohol.

Beer (12 ounces):
    Regular: 1 carb serving
    Light: ¼ to ½ carb serving
Sake (6 ounces): ⅔ carb serving
Wine (5 ounces):
    Champagne, brut: ⅓ carb serving
    Champagne, rosé: ¾ carb serving
    Red, dry: ⅓ carb serving
    White, dry: ⅓ carb serving
    White, sweet or dessert: 1 carb serving

(continued on next page)

Spirits (1½ ounces) = negligible carb servings

    Bourbon

    Brandy

    Cognac

    Gin

    Rum

    Scotch

    Tequila

    Vodka

    Whiskey

Caution: It's best to skip mixers, simple syrups, and liqueurs (like Campari, Cointreau, triple sec, or crème de anything) because these have a higher carb content; you'll be much better off going with club soda and adding fresh lemon or lime to your cocktails instead.

FOOD LABEL CLIFFS NOTES

You can also find carb price tags on packaged-food labels, though, of course, they're not labeled as such (that would just be *too* helpful). You'll need to do a smidge of detective work since they're expressed as grams of carbohydrates. To crack the code, remember this:

Approximately 15 grams of carbohydrates equals one serving of carbs, 30 grams equals two servings, and 45 grams equals three. Look first at the total carbohydrates listing on the nutrition facts panel to see what the item will add up to in terms of carb servings, based on that code. Next, look at the serving size at the top of the panel: While some packaged items may seem like only one serving, they may contain two or more.

It's also wise to check out the ingredients list, because what's in the food must be listed in descending order by weight (which means the highest amounts come first). This is handy to know so you can determine if sugar or other sweeteners are getting top billing (they'd be listed in the first few ingredients); the same is true for inflammation-triggering trans fats (which sometimes go by "partially hydrogenated oil") or other less desirable fats (like corn, soy, sunflower, safflower, and canola oil).

My advice is to also ditch anything with Splenda and other artificial sweeteners that contain a synthetic chemical called sucralose, which is 600 times sweeter than natural sugar (*seriously*). Because it's so much sweeter, you can end up over-stimulating your taste buds and actually change the way your taste buds perceive sweetness. Besides making you crave intensely sweet foods on the regular, this also somewhat desensitizes you to naturally sweet things. True story: I once had a Splenda-addicted client who needed to sprinkle at least one yellow packet on *fruit* because it simply didn't taste sweet enough for her in its natural state. So while using Splenda may cut down on your sugar intake in the short term, it also saddles you with an out-of-control sweet tooth. *Not worth it.*

Keep in mind: I don't recommend measuring out all your food (*who has the time or patience for that?*) but it can help for the first few days to get a visual of what, for instance, ⅓ cup cooked quinoa looks like (spoiler alert: It's probably significantly tinier than you think). That said, if you struggle with a Craving for Control, you may be better off skipping this step, to avoid fueling your natural tendency toward rigidity. After that, you can eyeball servings to see if they're on target and you can mix and match with ease. Once you have a basic understanding of the recommended carb servings, do yourself a favor and skip the math. One reason I love this plan so much is because it frees people up from calorie counting and general overthinking. If you follow these guidelines, there's really no need to count calories because you'll start resetting your hormones and your internal hunger and fullness cues. Remember, though, not all carbs are created equal: Serving for serving, some carb-rich foods (like fiber-packed sweet potatoes) are more nutritious than others (like bagels).

Once you have an idea of what the carb servings look like, you may find yourself jumping ahead and thinking about how many servings you tend to eat throughout the day. Great call, because after my clients and I discuss their food histories, that's our next step. If you're like most of my clients, you may find that, despite your best efforts, you may be eating well over five or six servings of carbs thanks to faux-healthy foods like granola, jelly and jam, excess fruit, and acai bowls, not to mention the sneaky sources of added sugar we talked about in the last chapter. *Don't panic.* Things are going to get easier from here on out.

The beauty of this approach is it gives you flexibility (as in: serious wiggle room) and helps you plan ahead. For instance, if you know you're going out for sushi for dinner, you could play it a couple of different ways: You could go lighter on the carbs at dinner with two pieces of sushi (around 1 carb serving), with the rest sashimi, a side of avocado, and a heaping handful of edamame (around 1 carb serving), in which case you could plan to eat two carb servings at breakfast, one carb serving at lunch, with low-carb snacks in the afternoon; *or*, if you're set on getting a 6-to-8-piece roll (which has 2 to 2½ carb servings), a couple pieces of nigiri, plus edamame and perhaps some sake, you could in theory just forfeit the majority of your carb servings earlier in the day, and focus on one really high-quality slow-burn carb serving for breakfast or lunch, along with leafy greens, ample fat, and protein. I don't actually recommend making this a nightly habit, though, because between the rice and the alcohol you are looking at a serious insulin surge. But this shows you how you can maintain flexibility and roll with the punches; it just requires some planning and some swaps. (You can factor in regular servings of chocolate this way, too.) In the next chapter, you'll find sample meal plans for Phase I so you can see how to put all of this into practice.

Ultimately, there's power in knowing the carb-swap system because it helps you prioritize the foods you want and make conscious, informed choices day in and day out. This way, you can stay flexible with your approach and make it work for you for the long haul. The plan is meant to help you stay accountable to yourself so you can decide what's worth spending your carb budget on. Personally, I wouldn't choose to splurge on fruit juice or jam because I'd much rather spend that carb cash on dark chocolate anything and sweet potato fries—but you may. You're in the driver's seat, so you get to decide how you want to divvy up your carb cash. There's no right or wrong approach, no one-size-fits-all answer—and that's why this plan works. It's geared toward getting your hormones working for you and helping you reclaim trust in your appetite. But just as important, this plan is reality-based so it's not something you can fall off of, regardless of the eating obstacles you've faced in the past.

Let's be real: I don't expect you to stay within your carb budget 24/7. Even with all the tools you've honed so far, occasional overeating is to be expected. So you can skip the guilt trip and just get right back to your carb-cash budgeting system with actual (and delicious) foods. You'll see how to put all these pieces together in the next chapter.

7

Become Your Own Sous-Chef (Mouthwatering Recipes Supplied)

A few years ago I read a "What's in Their Fridge?" magazine article featuring a busy restaurant chef and it kind of changed my life. I was initially intrigued because I assumed she would have an expert condiment collection—what I imagined might be an assortment of impossible-to-find fermented hot sauces, gourmet relishes, and international spice blends that maybe I'd consider buying in bulk for future housewarming gifts and then forget about. But what I discovered was *way* better. This chef had gone heavy on *mise-en-place*, one of the first lessons taught in culinary school, which literally means "put in place." It's a fancy phrase for a simple concept: having all your ingredients prepped and ready to go before you start cooking. Admittedly, it can seem a touch fussy, especially for home cooks, but I'm fairly certain that any professional chef would agree that it's one of the most crucial elements for cooking efficiently, wherever you are. Instead of rows of niche mustards and kimchi, this chef had containers of blanched asparagus and green beans, washed and dried lettuces, peeled onion and garlic, cooked brown rice, and a nice selection of proteins (including cooked chicken from what looked like last night's takeout). Her rationale: When she got home late from the restaurant, she was usually *famished*. After spending many hours making food for other people, this chef didn't want to make a big production for herself, but she also wasn't about to eat cereal for dinner. Her solution: precommitting to eating healthfully at home by being her own sous-chef.

Aside from achieving major fridge goals, what struck me most about this chef's approach was her relationship with food. The reality is, she has two: a professional one and a personal one. Cooking creative, delicious, aesthetically appealing meals for other people is literally her job; at the same time, she's a time-crunched woman in her early thirties who doesn't want to deny herself healthy, tasty meals. Her streamlined *mise-en-place* approach ensured that she didn't have to sacrifice her big-picture health goals, despite legitimate time challenges, because she had her prep down to a science. We could all take a page out of this chef's playbook. After all, besides being efficient, this practice helped her sidestep the hazards of post-work willpower depletion, when all bets are off.

Think about it: How many times have you intended to have

a much-needed date with a significant other, but then neither of you came up with a plan so you ended up hanging on the couch in sweats? Maybe that worked out okay and you enjoyed yourselves plenty (I hear you; there's arguably nobody who appreciates lounging more than me). But it's also possible that you later regretted missing an opportunity to put on real clothes for each other on a Saturday night. Similarly, how many times have you intended to cook a healthy meal after work but then thrown that plan out the window because you felt wiped out? Instead, you ordered not-so-healthy takeout or cobbled together what I like to call a sorority-girl special (some combination of cereal, crackers, and dip). As you know, it's pretty challenging to make healthy food choices in the throes of willpower depletion and decision fatigue (which affect most of us by around 3 or 4 p.m.). *This* is where sensible structure sans rigidity comes in.

Let me make something very clear: The goal isn't to go nuts with meal prepping *or* go full Barefoot Contessa every night (*although, how glorious would that be?*). But whether you want to cook regularly or be able to throw together an occasional lunch or dinner, the key to making non-meh meals in record time is thinking and *acting* ahead. In doing so, you can create no-brainer healthy, delicious meal-assembly plans (no complicated cooking required) for every meal. The first steps, as you saw in Chapter 5, are to plan ahead and stock the fridge and pantry with good-for-you baseline ingredients that you can use in the recipes that follow. The next step is to develop a prep plan that will work for you, which is what this chapter is all about.

This somewhat scrappy, assembly-style approach was borne out of necessity: Like most of my clients, I was too busy to cook…or so I thought. I would order delicious but very simple take-out meals, knowing that I could make them myself if I had the time, the inclination, and the right stuff on hand. Gradually, I became so fed up with the wait, the cost, and the texts behind this supposedly low-stress approach that I started getting inventive with using leftover chicken, salmon, or turkey and cobbling together balanced meals from there. As long as I had the protein, fresh veggies, a shallot or onion, and a flavorful sauce on hand, I didn't need to worry about concocting a creative meal at home. *Game changed.* I quickly discovered that light meal prep really works and is fairly painless. Don't get me wrong: I rarely prep *everything* for the week ahead of time. But I find that making a habit of having basic ingredients on hand not only gives me the opportunity to make delicious meals quickly, it also reduces stress and actually helps inspire creativity in the kitchen. If you spend an hour or so over the weekend to stock up and prep meal elements for the week ahead, your next-week self will be totally psyched.

PREP SCHOOL

The goal is to get ahead of the meal-prep challenge by buying or preparing what you can ahead of time. From the last few chapters, you probably have ideas for what should be on your shopping list; here, you'll learn how to put them all together. That said, it's best to think of the assembly meals that follow as *examples*, not rules. For instance, I love chicken and salmon and find them easy to prepare, so you'll see them frequently mentioned as potential protein options—but you may not feel the same way, and that's to be expected. You'll want to personalize your plan for *you* by thinking about your preferred sources of protein, and what sauces, veggie-based foundations, and fun additions (think nuts, seeds, onions, herbs, and spices) appeal to you. Don't stress about the details; you can modify these choices as you go along without driving yourself crazy doing all the prep that's outlined in the following recipes. But doing the basics to get your *mise-en-place* on—ricing cauliflower, spiralizing zucchini, preparing a spicy cabbage mix, making at least one sauce and buying organic rotisserie chicken or raw poultry for poaching—will make the coming week so much easier (and healthier) for you. If you don't feel like cooking all the proteins yourself, there are plenty of delicious, good-quality ones like organic rotisserie chicken, baked wild salmon fillets, even hard-boiled eggs, available at grocery stores. So cook what you can and want to, buy the rest, and do yourself a favor and cancel the guilt trip. What matters most is that you're stocked for the week.

In prepping ahead, the decision to eat healthfully throughout the week is already made for you. It's kind of like having a capsule wardrobe made up of super-versatile, mix-and-matchable pieces that you love wearing; only in this case, you'll have a well-edited selection of baseline ingredients that will facilitate kick-ass assembly-style meals in no time. By giving yourself a leg up on the prep process, you'll end up saving time instead of stressing in the kitchen; you'll also be preserving your valuable (and limited) self-control for times when you really need it. Let's face it: You won't always have the option to plan ahead; sometimes, you'll have to wing it because, hey, that's real life. Oh, and if you've never been fond of veggies, prepare to come around (to the green side). Between the salads drenched in savory full-fat dressings, zoodles smothered in robust sauces, and Brussels sprouts chips, I've converted more than a few stubborn naysayers—and I expect you'll join them.

IT'S ALL ABOUT THAT BASE

Let's kick things off at the same place steamy hook-up sessions unfold: first base. In this case, I'm talking about what will become the base for your meals for lunch and dinner. We're starting here because I find that people struggle most with what to eat for lunch and dinner, especially because as the day goes on, decision fatigue and willpower depletion start kicking in. (I promise we'll get to breakfast later.) Once you have your base prepared, launching into meal assembly is a breeze because the blueprint for meal assembly is this simple: **Base + flavorful sauce/dressing + protein of your choice.** And *voila*! Your meal is ready.

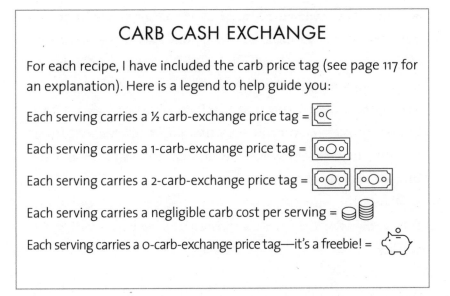

CARB CASH EXCHANGE

For each recipe, I have included the carb price tag (see page 117 for an explanation). Here is a legend to help guide you:

Each serving carries a ½ carb-exchange price tag =

Each serving carries a 1-carb-exchange price tag =

Each serving carries a 2-carb-exchange price tag =

Each serving carries a negligible carb cost per serving =

Each serving carries a 0-carb-exchange price tag—it's a freebie! =

Zucchini Noodles (Zoodles)

As a base, zucchini noodles (aka zoodles, zinguini, or spiral-ized zucchini) are a fairly big deal because they hold flavorful sauce really well and take less than 5 minutes to prepare. To make the thin strips of zucchini, you'll need a spiralizer, or you can find them pre-spiralized at many grocery stores. About 2 zucchini is a serving (although you're welcome to eat as much as your heart desires). I like to sauté the zucchini strands in olive oil or ghee with a pinch of sea salt for about 2 minutes before adding the sauce; this makes for extra–al dente "noodles." (I'd caution against overcooking them, since the zucchini will release a good amount of liquid when heated, and you don't want to end up with watery pasta.)

Kelp noodles, which are also great at holding flavorful sauces, but not quite as versatile in my opinion, work especially well with sesame tahini sauce and require little to no prep, which is especially clutch when you're in a pinch. Pair zoodles or kelp noodles with the four sauces that follow and 4 to 6 ounces of high-quality protein like poached chicken, store-bought rotisserie chicken, wild salmon, two eggs, or another protein of your choosing.

Similarly, you can prep the spicy cabbage mix and cauliflower rice ahead of time and use them as bases during the week.

Spicy Cabbage Mix

Makes about 10 cups; serves 4 to 6

Truth be told, this recipe was an accidental but welcome discovery: While testing recipes for my site in 2016, I found myself with *a lot* of leftover cabbage mix. At first, I wasn't sure what to do with the surplus, but I quickly realized that it goes with just about everything. This makes the raw veggie blend kind of the ultimate meal-assembly tool, plus it requires zero cooking; all you've got to do is pair it with a delicious, flavorful sauce, 4 to 6 ounces of protein, and fun additions like sesame seeds. Without question, it has become my lunch base of choice. (Note: I like shredding my carrots and serrano chile together in a food processor for maximum efficiency, but you can chop these finely by hand as well. For less heat, remove the ribs and seeds.)

1 head napa (or other) cabbage, sliced into ¼-inch-thick rounds

2 unpeeled carrots, chopped or shredded

1 serrano chile pepper, chopped or shredded

Put the cabbage in a large bowl. Blitz the carrots and chile in a food processor, then add them to the bowl. Mix the ingredients well and store in an airtight container in the fridge; it'll stay fresh for up to 5 days.

Cauliflower Rice Base

I'm completely in love with cauliflower rice, and I have a feeling you will be, too, once you incorporate these variations into your routine. As you'll see, it's super easy to make, but some grocery stores sell it pre-riced, and that absolutely works, too. If you're ricing your own cauliflower at home, it will keep in an airtight container in the fridge for up to 4 days.

VARIATION No. 1

CAULIFLOWER RICE, BIBIMBAP STYLE

Serves 2 to 3

Not yet a cauliflower rice convert? Prepare to become one. If you're adding shredded chicken, you'll want to toss it in when you mix in the scallions; alternatively, cooked eggs and salmon work great placed on top.

The "rice"

1 head cauliflower, cut into small florets, or 1 pound store-
    bought riced cauliflower
3 tablespoons extra-virgin olive oil
2 tablespoons coconut aminos
2 tablespoons brown rice vinegar
5 scallions (white part only), chopped (about ¼ cup)
Pinch of sea salt

The bibimbap

2 to 3 tablespoons hot sesame oil
2 to 3 tablespoons sesame seeds
½ carrot, julienned or sliced into matchsticks
½ cup kimchi

Pulse the cauliflower florets in a food processor until the pieces are
the size of couscous (you should have about 2 cups). Heat the olive
oil in a sauté pan over high heat. Add the cauliflower, coconut aminos, and vinegar, and sauté until the cauliflower starts to lightly
brown, 3 to 5 minutes. Stir in the scallions and salt to taste. Divide
into the desired servings and garnish with hot sesame oil, sesame
seeds, carrot, and kimchi.

CARB CASH EXCHANGE:

VARIATION NO. 2

CAULIFLOWER RICE, MEXI-CALI STYLE

Serves 2 to 3

I love this variation with shredded chicken for lunch and dinner, but I've also tried it as a breakfast dish with eggs and it did not disappoint. If you're adding shredded chicken, you'll want to add it when you mix in the lime juice, but cooked eggs and salmon work well when placed on top. For Phase II, feel free to add a serving of black beans.

The "rice"

1 head cauliflower, cut into small florets, or 1 pound store-bought riced cauliflower
3 tablespoons extra-virgin olive oil
1 cup chopped purple cabbage (about ¼ pound)
5 scallions (white part only), chopped (about ¼ cup)
1½ tablespoons fresh lime juice
Pinch of sea salt

The garnish

⅓ cup Garlic Crema Dressing (page 145)
1 avocado, pitted, peeled, and cubed
¼ cup salsa
1 tablespoon pepitas (optional)

Pulse the cauliflower florets in a food processor until the pieces are the size of couscous (you should have about 2 cups). Heat the oil in a sauté pan over high heat. Add the cauliflower, cabbage, scallions, and lime juice and sauté until the cauliflower starts to lightly brown, 3 to 5 minutes. Salt to taste. Divide into the desired servings and garnish with garlic crema, avocado, salsa, and pepitas.

CARB CASH EXCHANGE: 🪙🪙

VARIATION No. 3

CAULIFLOWER RICE, CURRY STYLE

Serves 2 to 3

This combo of savory spices makes for an extra-comforting, warming dish for cold nights.

The "rice"

1 head cauliflower, cut into small florets, or 1 pound store-bought riced cauliflower

2 to 3 tablespoons ghee

1 cup snap peas

½ bell pepper, seeded, de-ribbed, and thinly sliced (about ½ cup)

The garnish

¼ cup Curry in a Hurry sauce (page 144)

¼ cup roasted cashews

Pulse the cauliflower florets in a food processor until the pieces are the size of couscous (you should have about 2 cups). Melt the ghee in a sauté pan over high heat. Add the cauliflower and sauté until it starts to lightly brown, 3 to 5 minutes. Add the snap peas and bell pepper and sauté for 1 minute. Divide into the desired servings and garnish with the curry sauce and cashews.

CARB CASH EXCHANGE: [image: bill icon] (if you divide the recipe into two servings)

VARIATION No. 4

MULTITASKING CAULIFLOWER BASE

Makes 6 to 8 (3- to 4-inch) tortillas, or 1 large pizza crust; serves 2 to 3

I'm *deep* into cauliflower right now. (*Can you tell?*) This base requires the most legwork of the four, but it makes for an ultra-versatile vehicle for delicious toppings. In fact, it can be used as a pizza crust, tortillas for tacos, or an alternative bread-type-thing for avocado "toast." The cauliflower pizza crust is incredible with Epic Vegetable Bolognese (page 142) or the Simple Pesto Sauce (page 142), topped with poached chicken and Rustic Roasted Mushrooms (page 169). I'm also obsessed with the cauliflower tortillas paired with the Spicy Cabbage Mix (page 134) and Garlic Crema Dressing (page 145) along with shredded chicken or salmon. If you're making tacos for Phase I, feel free to add ⅓ cup quinoa for a 1-carb serving, and for Phase II, you can add ½ cup black beans for a 1-carb serving.

1 head cauliflower, cut into small florets, or 1 pound store-bought riced cauliflower

2 eggs

Pinch of sea salt

Optional seasonings

Red pepper flakes and nutritional yeast (for pizza crust)

Grated zest of ½ lime (for tortillas and toast)

Preheat the oven to 375°F and line a baking sheet with parchment paper. Pulse the florets in a food processor until the pieces are the size of couscous (you should have about 2 cups). Put the riced cauliflower in a steamer basket and steam over boiling water in a covered saucepan for 5 minutes, then let cool. Place the steamed cauliflower in a square of cheesecloth or a nut milk bag and squeeze out as much of the excess liquid as you can; otherwise, you'll end up with a soggy crust or soggy tortillas, so put some forearm muscle into it and make it count. Transfer the drained cauliflower to a bowl and mix in the eggs, salt, and optional seasonings. On the prepared baking sheet, spread the mixture evenly into a large, fairly flat round for a pizza crust, or 6 to 8 smaller rounds or squares for tortillas or toast. Bake for 8 to 10 minutes, then flip (carefully) and cook for another 7 to 9 minutes, or until golden.

CARB CASH EXCHANGE:

My Secret Sauces

Sometimes, welcoming a new sauce or dressing into the rotation is all it takes to bring your meal game up a notch. These recipes are my secret weapons when it comes to eating well, especially when time is scarce, because they can take very healthy but otherwise ordinary foods like plain veggies and poached chicken and turn them into ridiculously tasty, satisfying dishes in a matter of seconds. Robust full-fat, flavorful sauces and dressings are the key to creating meal-assembly dishes you actually want to eat. Best of all, the multitasking sauces that follow can be matched with different bases and protein choices, providing built-in variety to your meals.

Tahini Sauce

Makes about ¾ cup; serves 3

This creamy sauce is delicious on zoodles and kelp noodles with cooked chicken or a sunny-side-up egg. I love topping this dish with toasted sesame seeds and scallions. Bonus: Any leftover sauce is incredible as a makeshift satay dip for chicken.

½ cup tahini
2 cloves garlic
1-inch piece fresh ginger, peeled
2 tablespoons coconut aminos
1 tablespoon brown rice vinegar
1 teaspoon hot sesame oil

Blitz all the ingredients in a high-speed blender until smooth. Store in an airtight container in the fridge for up to 1 week.

CARB CASH EXCHANGE: [°C per ¼ cup serving of sauce

Simple Pesto Sauce

Makes about 1 cup; serves 3 to 4

This sauce is one of the most versatile in the mix. You can use it on pretty much anything savory, from zoodles or kelp noodles (with chicken and freshly sliced tomato) to Cauliflower Pizza Crust (page 139) and Baked Frittata Muffins (page 156). Or, you can enjoy it as a stand-alone dipping sauce for crudités.

2 cloves garlic, chopped
1 tablespoon tahini
1 cup lightly packed fresh basil leaves
Grated zest and juice of ½ lemon
½ cup unsalted roasted pistachios
½ cup extra-virgin olive oil
Sea salt

Blend the garlic, tahini, basil, lemon zest and juice, pistachios, and olive oil in a high-speed blender until smooth. Season to taste with salt. Store in an airtight container in the fridge for up to 1 week.

CARB CASH EXCHANGE:

Epic Vegetable Bolognese

Makes 5½ cups; serves 7 (about ¾ cup per serving)

This recipe was inspired by my dear friend Laurel Gallucci, of Sweet Laurel Bakery. It's hard to believe this sauce is dairy-free, because its creaminess suggests otherwise. The prep is a bit more time-consuming than that of the other sauces, but trust me: It's worth it. Plus, this recipe makes a large quantity that can be frozen. Pro tip: I love freezing mine in silicone ice-cube trays for easy access and speedier defrosting. I live for this bolognese on zoodles with chicken (or sautéed ground grass-fed lamb), but it also works really well on a cauliflower pizza crust as an exceptionally hearty tomato sauce.

¼ cup extra-virgin olive oil

1 onion, chopped

3 unpeeled carrots, chopped

2 large leeks (white and light green parts), chopped

2 cloves garlic

2 portobello mushrooms, sliced

2 tablespoons apple cider vinegar

1 (26.5-ounce) box crushed tomatoes

1 teaspoon sea salt

½ cup pine nuts

In a Dutch oven or other heavy pot, heat the olive oil over medium-high heat. Add the onion, carrots, leeks, garlic, and mushrooms and sauté for 15 minutes, or until the onion starts to caramelize. Add the vinegar and tomatoes and sauté for 10 minutes, stirring constantly. Add the salt. In batches, purée the sauce in a high-speed blender and empty into a storage container; add the pine nuts to the last batch and blend at high speed until smooth. Stir into the puréed sauce in the container. Store in an airtight container in the fridge for up to 1 week or freeze in an ice cube tray for up to 3 months.

CARB CASH EXCHANGE: 🪙🪙

Curry in a Hurry

Makes about ½ cup; serves 2

This rich, fragrant curry sauce is perfect on zoodles or kelp noodles (with chicken or another protein), and even better when topped with a handful of roasted cashews. It's also delicious on cauliflower rice with sugar snap peas and sliced bell pepper. I like this dish extra spicy, but if you're not looking for a ton of heat, feel free to dial down the quantity of curry paste.

 2 tablespoons ghee
 1 clove garlic, minced or grated
 1 tablespoon grated fresh ginger
 1 tablespoon plus 1 teaspoon red curry paste
 1 cup full-fat coconut milk
 1 tablespoon fresh lime juice
 1 tablespoon fish sauce

Melt the ghee in a saucepan over medium-low heat. Add the garlic, ginger, and curry paste, stirring constantly for about 30 seconds. Add the coconut milk, lime juice, and fish sauce and increase the heat to high to bring the sauce to a boil. Cook for 3 to 5 minutes, or until fragrant, stirring constantly. Serve warm or store in an airtight container in the fridge for up to 1 week.

CARB CASH EXCHANGE: $\boxed{\circ\bigcirc\circ}$ per ¼ cup serving

GARLIC CREMA DRESSING

Makes about ½ cup; serves 2

Hands down easiest-ever dressing! I love a salad made with Spicy Cabbage Mix (page 134), this dressing, poached chicken, sliced avocado, sliced tomatoes, and pepitas. Karam's Garlic Sauce (page 85) is my all-time favorite condiment and best-kept secret (until now!) because it tastes like the old-school ranch dressing of my youth, sans dairy. It's the backbone to many of my salad dressings and marinades, and I also love it for dipping crudités.

   ⅓ cup Karam's Garlic Sauce (page 85)
   Juice of ½ lemon

Whisk together the garlic sauce and lemon juice. This will keep well in a covered jar in the fridge for up to 1 week.

CARB CASH EXCHANGE:

CHINESE CHICKEN SALAD DRESSING

Makes about ½ cup; serves 2

Traditional Chinese chicken salad dressings are often loaded with so much sugar that they taste a bit like dessert. This one manages to come in really strong with only some naturally occurring sweetness from the cashews and coconut aminos. I highly recommend pairing this rich, tangy dressing with Spicy Cabbage Mix (page 134), poached chicken or salmon, sliced avocado, sliced scallions, and toasted sesame seeds for a next-level delicious salad.

   3 tablespoons extra-virgin olive oil
   1½ tablespoons brown rice vinegar
   1½ tablespoons coconut aminos
   2 tablespoons unsweetened cashew butter
   1 teaspoon hot toasted sesame oil

Whisk together all the ingredients. Store in a jar or bottle in the fridge for up to 1 week.

CARB CASH EXCHANGE: ⬚ per ¼ cup serving

SPICY THAI DRESSING

Makes about ⅓ cup; serves 2

Tangy, salty, and spicy—personally, I love this one with Spicy Cabbage Mix (page 134), poached chicken or fish, toasted cashews, sliced scallions, and toasted sesame seeds.

   Grated zest of ½ lime
   ¼ cup lime juice
   2 tablespoons fish sauce
   1 tablespoon brown rice vinegar
   1 tablespoon coconut aminos
   1 tablespoon hot sesame oil

Whisk together all the ingredients. Store in a jar or bottle in the fridge for up to 1 week.

CARB CASH EXCHANGE: ⬤⬚

Turmeric Tahini Sauce

Makes about ¾ cup; serves 2 to 3

When I was in grad school in NYC, I found safe haven at an uber-crunchy café that was hidden inside a yoga studio. The place is called Jivamukti, and it serves the type of food you'd expect to find at a crunchy yoga studio café—except for the turmeric tahini, which is otherworldly. When I moved back to LA I found myself missing that sauce so much that I decided to concoct my own version.

½ cup tahini
¼ cup lemon juice
1 tablespoon water
1 tablespoon coconut aminos
2 cloves garlic
1 teaspoon ground turmeric
¼ teaspoon sea salt
¼ teaspoon paprika

Blitz all the ingredients in a high-speed blender until smooth. Store in an airtight container in the fridge for up to 1 week.

CARB CASH EXCHANGE:

Lemon-Herb Vinaigrette

Makes about ⅓ cup; serves 2

This one's a nod to one of my favorite salads of all time from the Los Angeles resto The Sycamore Kitchen. I've never managed to get them to spill the beans on their recipe, but this is my take; it's not quite the same but it comes close enough. I love this dressing on an Italian-style chopped salad (my go-to Sycamore order) with kale, cabbage, radicchio, chicken, roasted nuts (Spicy Mixed Nuts on page 162 work great here), and tomatoes.

> Juice of ½ lemon
> ¼ cup extra-virgin olive oil
> 1 tablespoon apple cider vinegar
> 1½ shallots
> Leaves from 1 sprig fresh rosemary
> Leaves from 1 sprig fresh thyme
> Sea salt and pepper

Blitz the lemon juice, olive oil, vinegar, shallots, rosemary, and thyme in a high-speed blender until smooth. Season with salt and pepper to taste. Store in an airtight container in the fridge for up to 1 week.

CARB CASH EXCHANGE:

Rustic Apple Cider Mustard Dressing

Makes about ⅓ cup; serves 2

This one works especially well on a simple fall-*ish* salad with protein and roasted walnuts. Orange-Rosemary Pecans (page 164) also are delish with this.

6 tablespoons extra-virgin olive oil

2 tablespoons apple cider vinegar

2 teaspoons whole-grain mustard

Leaves from 1 sprig fresh rosemary

Leaves from 1 sprig fresh thyme

2 oil-packed anchovies

Blitz all the ingredients in a high-speed blender until smooth. Store in an airtight container in the fridge for up to 3 days.

CARB CASH EXCHANGE:

Garlic–White Wine Vinaigrette

Makes about ½ cup; serves 2 to 3

This one is an all-time family favorite in my house. It's incredible on a simple salad as well as drizzled over salmon.

¼ cup extra virgin-olive oil

2 heaping tablespoons Majestic Garlic Spread (see Pantry Essentials)

2 tablespoons white wine vinegar

Pinch of sea salt

Whisk together all the ingredients. Store in an airtight container in the fridge for up to 1 week.

CARB CASH EXCHANGE:

VARIATION ON A CLASSIC

POACHED CHICKEN

Serves 4

Once cooked, this tender chicken can be shredded for tacos, sautéed with zoodles, used in a cauliflower-rice bowl or stir-fry, or placed in a well-dressed salad. I learned this old-school technique from beloved LA cooking teacher Pamela Salzman and do it nearly every Sunday. (Note: Fresh garlic and chopped onion also work in this recipe, but this is the down-and-dirty version I make at home.)

 4 bone-in, skin-on chicken legs or breasts
 ¼ cup kosher salt (to flavor the water)
 Garlic powder
 Onion powder

Put the chicken in a pot with the salt, a couple dashes of garlic and onion powder (see Note), and enough water to cover by 1 inch. Bring the water to a boil over high heat, then reduce the heat to low, cover, and simmer for about 25 minutes, or until the chicken is cooked through. (That means a meat thermometer will register an internal temperature of 165 degrees and the juices will run clear.) Let the chicken cool in the poaching liquid for about 25 minutes. I love roasted chicken skin, but I'm not so fond of the texture of poached chicken skin so I remove it (but that's your call). Shred or slice the chicken meat off the bone and keep it in an airtight container in the fridge for up to 1 week. (You might want to save the poaching liquid in an airtight container in the fridge to use as broth within the next couple of days.)

Now that you have all the necessary building blocks to assemble truly satisfying meals throughout the week, it's time to think about how you might put the pieces together. I could spend a whole paragraph (or two or three) walking you through the drill, but that might make it seem more complicated than it needs to be. This is a scenario in which a visual aid is worth more than a bunch of text—because the formula really is *that* simple. So here's the deal:

HOW TO
BUILD A ZOODLE BOWL

Choose your:

① Base	② Protein	③ Sauce / Dressing	+ The Fun Stuff
zoodles	4 to 6 ounces poached or rotisserie chicken	Tahini Sauce (page 141)	A DOSE OF HEAT hot sesame oil, chile peppers, minced ginger

(continued on next page)

① Base	② Protein	③ Sauce / Dressing	+ The Fun Stuff
kelp noodles	4 to 6 ounces cooked turkey, lamb, or bison	Simple Pesto Sauce (page 142)	ROASTED NUTS + SEEDS toasted sesame seeds, cashews, pine nuts
	4 to 6 ounces cooked salmon or cod	Epic Vegetable Bolognese (page 142)	ONION FAMILY thinly sliced scallions, garlic, shallot, chives
	2 eggs	Curry in a Hurry (page 144)	FRESH HERBS rosemary, thyme, mint, basil

HOW TO
BUILD A SPICY CABBAGE MIX SALAD

Choose your:

① Base	② Protein	③ Sauce / Dressing	+ The Fun Stuff
Spicy Cabbage Mix (page 134)	4 to 6 ounces poached or rotisserie chicken	Garlic Crema Dressing (page 145)	A DOSE OF HEAT ginger, cayenne, paprika, cumin, sliced chiles

	4 to 6 ounces cooked turkey, lamb, or bison	Chinese Chicken Salad Dressing (page 145)	ROASTED NUTS + SEEDS toasted sesame seeds, cashews
	4 to 6 ounces cooked salmon or cod	Spicy Thai Dressing (page 146)	ONION FAMILY thinly sliced scallions, garlic, shallot, chives
	2 eggs		FRESH HERBS cilantro, mint, basil
			SOUR sauerkraut, kimchi
			CREAMY avocado
			UMAMI coconut aminos, nori, furikake

HOW TO
BUILD A CAULIFLOWER-RICE BOWL

Choose your:

1 Base	**2** Protein	**3** Sauce / Dressing	**+** The Fun Stuff
Cauliflower rice (page 135)	Mexi-Cali style: 4 to 6 ounces poached or rotisserie chicken	Garlic Crema Dressing (page 145)	A DOSE OF HEAT ginger, cayenne, paprika, cumin, sliced chiles, salsa

(continued on next page)

① Base	② Protein	③ Sauce / Dressing	+ The Fun Stuff
	Bibimbap style: 4 to 6 ounces cooked turkey, lamb, or bison	coconut aminos + rice vinegar + hot sesame oil	ROASTED NUTS + SEEDS pepitas, toasted sesame seeds, cashews
	4 to 6 ounces cooked salmon or cod	Curry in a Hurry (page 144)	ONION FAMILY thinly sliced scallions, garlic, shallot, chives
	2 eggs		FRESH HERBS cilantro, mint, basil
			SOUR sauerkraut, kimchi
			CREAMY avocado
			UMAMI coconut aminos, nori, furikake

HOW TO
BUILD ON A CAULIFLOWER CRUST

Choose your:

①\newline Base	②\newline Protein	③\newline Sauce /\newline Dressing	+\newline The Fun\newline Stuff
Cauliflower crust (page 139)	**pizza**\newline 4 to 6 ounces poached or rotisserie chicken	Simple Pesto Sauce (page 142)\newline or\newline Epic Vegetable Bolognese (page 142)	A DOSE OF HEAT\newline red pepper flakes, cayenne, paprika, cumin, sliced chiles, salsa
	tacos\newline 4 to 6 ounces cooked turkey, lamb, or bison	Garlic Crema Dressing (page 145)	ROASTED NUTS + SEEDS\newline toasted pine nuts, hemp seeds, pepitas
	4 to 6 ounces cooked salmon or cod		ONION FAMILY\newline thinly sliced onion, garlic, shallot, leek
	2 eggs		FRESH HERBS\newline basil, sun-dried tomatoes, cilantro
			SOUR\newline lime, sauerkraut, kimchi
			CREAMY\newline Avocado

HOW TO GET CREATIVE

Here's the thing: Now that you've gotten a feel for how to assemble a tasty "divvy up"–style meal, there's no need to color within the lines of specific mix-and-match variations I've laid out in this chapter. In fact, I totally encourage you to play around with things like cauliflower rice, zoodles, and roasted veggies, adding your own personal touches. The same goes for your sources of protein. If you're a pescatarian, you'll want to ditch the chicken and experiment with different types of fish and seafood. These meals are meant to act as a blueprint that you can fill in based on your personal faves, tastes, and preferences.

Prep School: Breakfast

All these tasty breakfast options can be prepped at least partly ahead of time, requiring little to no effort in the a.m.

BAKED FRITTATA MUFFINS

Makes 12 egg muffins; serves 4

My busy mom clients are often exceptionally short on time, especially in the morning, so I originally developed this protein-packed, make-ahead recipe for them. Getting out the door is hard enough, so I wanted to give them something they could realistically throw together ahead of time but is also really delish and versatile. These frittata muffins can be paired with a handful of the recipes in this chapter from Simple Pesto Sauce (page 142) to Rustic Roasted Mushrooms (page 169) and Brussels Sprouts Chips (page 164).

  12 eggs
  Sea salt and pepper
  ¼ cup extra-virgin olive oil
  3 portobello mushrooms, chopped
  1 leek (white and light green parts), chopped
  1 white onion, chopped

Preheat the oven to 425°F and prepare a silicone, lined, or greased (with olive or avocado oil) 12-cup muffin tin. In a large bowl, beat the eggs and season with salt and pepper. In a sauté pan, heat the oil over medium-high heat. Add the mushrooms, leek, and onion and cook, stirring frequently, until the vegetables have released their liquid and are lightly browned, 9 to 11 minutes. Transfer the mushroom mixture to the eggs and mix well. Distribute evenly in the muffin cups. Bake for 15 to 18 minutes, or until a toothpick comes out clean. (Note: I recommend placing the muffin pan on a baking tray for easy transfer and spill prevention.) Store in an airtight container in the fridge for up to 4 days.

CARB CASH EXCHANGE:

RASPBERRY BARS

Makes 6 bars; serves 6

I originally made a layered-dessert variation of these bars for my site and ended up eating the leftover slivers for breakfast the next morning. Unfortunately, the slivers were a bit small for a legit meal, and a full bar was too sweet for breakfast, so I re-jiggered the recipe and dialed down the carbs considerably so it could work as a not-just-for-special-occasions breakfast. I almost couldn't believe it—this version is just as good. (Note: Psyllium husk is a great flavorless fiber that acts like a thickening agent to bind the raspberry mixture. You can find it at most natural foods stores or online. It's not essential, especially as far as taste goes, but it makes the raspberry layer hold together better.)

The crust

1 cup almond or hazelnut flour
½ cup coconut oil, melted
¼ cup maple syrup
1 teaspoon vanilla extract
Pinch of sea salt

The filling

4 cups fresh raspberries
2 tablespoons psyllium husk
Grated zest and juice of ½ lemon, plus more zest for garnish

Preheat the oven to 350°F. Line a shallow baking dish with parchment paper (I use an 8-by-10-inch baking dish that's 2 inches deep). Put the nut flour, coconut oil, maple syrup, vanilla extract, and salt in a food processor or high-speed blender and pulse until a thick paste forms. Evenly spread the mixture in the prepared pan. Put the filling ingredients in a food processor or high-speed blender and pulse or blend until it reaches a creamy consistency. Pour the filling over the crust and smooth it with a spatula. Bake for 25 minutes. Remove the dish from the oven, let it cool completely, then chill in the fridge until firm, about 30 minutes. Top with additional lemon zest and cut into 6 bars. Store in an airtight container in the fridge for up to a week.

CARB CASH EXCHANGE: 〔∘O∘〕 〔∘C per bar

SUPER-SIMPLE SMOOTHIE

Serves 1

This is my busy-morning breakfast of choice because it's quick and kind of tastes like cookie dough. I like to add two scoops of unsweetened vanilla collagen protein powder; you could also add something like hemp seeds or spirulina for added protein, if you want. (Note: I like using a silicone ice tray to freeze the coconut milk.)

½ cup full-fat coconut milk, frozen (see Note, above)
½ cup water
1 medjool date, pitted
¼ teaspoon matcha
Pinch of sea salt

Combine all the ingredients in a high-speed blender and blitz until smooth.

CARB CASH EXCHANGE: 〔∘O∘〕 〔∘O∘〕

CHIA SEED PUDDING

Serves 1

It's delicious, easy on the carb cash—and what's better than making breakfast while you sleep?

   1 cup full-fat coconut milk
   ¼ cup chia seeds
   1 tablespoon unsweetened almond butter
   1 teaspoon maple syrup
   ½ teaspoon vanilla extract
   Pinch of ground cinnamon
   Pinch of sea salt

Combine all the ingredients in a bowl or jar and mix well, making sure the almond butter and chia seeds are evenly distributed. Cover and refrigerate overnight. This pudding will keep for up to 3 days covered in the fridge.

CARB CASH EXCHANGE: [○◯○]

"BUTTERMILK" PANCAKES

Makes 8 to 10 (4-inch) pancakes; serves 3

Okay, fine, this isn't necessarily a make-ahead recipe, but these pancakes are so delish, satisfying, and perfect for a cozy, lazy Sunday morning.

1 large egg

¾ cup coconut milk

1 tablespoon lemon juice

2 tablespoons coconut oil or ghee, melted, plus more for the skillet

¼ cup water

1½ cups almond or hazelnut flour

½ cup tapioca starch

½ teaspoon baking powder

½ teaspoon baking soda

½ teaspoon sea salt

Whisk together the egg, coconut milk, lemon juice, oil or ghee, and water. Stir the dry ingredients together in a bowl with a whisk. Fold in the wet ingredients, adding water if the batter looks too dry. Heat a skillet over medium-high heat and coat it with coconut oil or ghee. Ladle in as many pancakes as can fit comfortably. (Note: I like ladling the batter in with a ¼-cup measuring cup, filled three-fourths full.) Cook the pancakes for about 2 minutes, or until bubbles appear on the surface. Flip them and cook for about 1 minute on the other side, or until they're golden brown. Repeat the process until you run out of batter. Before serving, feel free to top the pancakes with ghee or nut butter and cinnamon.

CARB CASH EXCHANGE: ⌐○○○⌐ ⌐○○○⌐ per three pancakes

MAKE-AHEAD MULTITASKING SNACKS

Sometimes snacking gets a bad rap, and that's because between-meal noshing in the throes of willpower depletion often means indulging in excess sweet or salty starches. But snacking has a well-deserved place in a healthy-eating plan because it can really help manage your appetite, keep energy steady, and prevent *hangry* outbursts. So kick any residual snacking guilt to the curb and precommit to keeping these delicious snacks on hand.

SPICY MIXED NUTS

Makes 1 cup; serves 4

If I'm being honest, a plain, unsalted raw nut does absolutely nothing for me. But a roasted spicy nut? Now we're talking! These flavorful mixed nuts are great for snacking, and they're an incredible addition to Cauliflower Rice, Mexi-Cali Style (page 137). Feel free to switch up the types of nuts you use, or you can opt to stick with one of your favorite nuts instead of a combo.

- ⅓ cup raw pecans
- ⅓ cup raw walnuts
- ⅓ cup raw pepitas
- 1 tablespoon extra-virgin olive oil
- 1 teaspoon garlic powder
- 1 teaspoon onion powder
- ½ teaspoon paprika, plus more for garnish
- ¼ teaspoon cayenne
- ¼ teaspoon sea salt

Preheat the oven to 350°F and line a baking sheet with parchment paper. Toss the nuts with olive oil and spices on the prepared baking sheet. Roast for 12 to 15 minutes or until golden, flipping once.

Top with additional paprika to taste. These will stay fresh in an air-tight container in the fridge for a week.

CARB CASH EXCHANGE:

Maple-Sesame Cashews

Makes 1 cup; serves 4

When I'm looking for a snack that's a little sweet and a little salty, I grab these cashews. They taste kind of like pasteli, the thin little Middle Eastern sesame seed candies I was obsessed with as a kid.

- 1 cup raw cashews
- 2 tablespoons coconut aminos
- 1 tablespoon coconut oil, melted
- 2 teaspoons maple syrup
- 1 teaspoon coconut sugar
- ½ teaspoon vanilla extract
- ¼ teaspoon sea salt
- 1 tablespoon unsweetened shredded coconut
- 1 tablespoon sesame seeds

Preheat the oven to 350°F and line a baking sheet with parchment paper. Toss the nuts with the coconut aminos, coconut oil, maple syrup, coconut sugar, vanilla extract, and salt on the prepared baking sheet. Top with shredded coconut and sesame seeds. Roast for 12 to 15 minutes, or until golden, flipping once. These will stay fresh in an airtight container in the fridge for 1 week.

CARB CASH EXCHANGE: per ¼ cup serving

Orange-Rosemary Pecans

Makes 1 cup; serves 4

To me, these pecans taste like fall: warm, rich, and savory. They're a great topping for salads, especially with the Rustic Apple Cider Mustard Dressing on page 148.

> 1 cup raw pecans
> Juice of 1 small orange (I love blood oranges but any type works)
> 1 tablespoon coconut oil, melted
> Leaves from 2 sprigs fresh rosemary
> Leaves from 2 sprigs fresh thyme
> ½ teaspoon ground cumin
> ¼ teaspoon sea salt
> Grated zest of 1 small orange, plus more for garnish

Preheat the oven to 350°F and line a baking sheet with parchment paper. Toss the pecans with the orange juice, coconut oil, rosemary, thyme, cumin, and salt on the prepared baking sheet. Roast for 12 to 15 minutes or until golden, flipping once. Top with orange zest to taste. These will stay fresh in an airtight container in the fridge for a week.

CARB CASH EXCHANGE: 🗒️ per ¼ cup serving

Brussels Sprouts Chips

Makes 1 cup; serves 2

These offer all the salty, crunchy goodness of a regular chip, without the heavy carb price tag. This recipe calls for half a pound of

Brussels sprouts, but you'll only be using the *outer* leaves because they crisp up way better than the inner ones. Don't worry about the inner leaves going to waste: They work great sautéed in omelets and in Baked Frittata Muffins (page 156), or use them as a topping for cauliflower-rice bowls.

Outer leaves of ½ pound Brussels sprouts (about 12 sprouts), about 2 cups

3 to 4 tablespoons extra-virgin olive oil

Pinch of sea salt

1 teaspoon garlic powder

1 teaspoon onion powder

Preheat the oven to 350°F and line a baking sheet with parchment paper. Toss the leaves with the olive oil and spices on the prepared baking sheet. Roast for 15 minutes, or until golden, flipping once. Remove from the oven and let the chips cool completely on the baking sheet. You can store these in an airtight container in a cool, dry place for up to 3 days.

CARB CASH EXCHANGE: 🪙🪙

Chocolate-Orange Energy Bites

Makes 10 small bites; serves 5

Energy bites are great for those times when you're looking for a lot of flavor in a portable little package. This version tastes like a not-so-sweet chocolate-orange truffle. *Enough said.*

½ cup raw pecans

6 medjool dates, pitted

2½ tablespoons unsweetened raw cacao powder

Grated zest of ½ orange

⅛ teaspoon sea salt

In a high-speed blender or a food processor, combine all the ingredients and blend until smooth. Use your hands to form the mixture into 10 balls (about 1 inch in diameter). Refrigerate until firm, about 30 minutes. Serve chilled. These will stay fresh in an airtight container in the fridge for up to 1 week.

CARB CASH EXCHANGE: [∘O∘] per bite

LEMON–POPPY SEED BITES

Makes 10 small bites; serves 5

These bite-sized snacks taste like lemon–poppy seed cookie dough: sweet, zesty, and fresh. Unlike cookie dough, they're healthful. They're even a great grab-and-go option for breakfast.

½ cup cashews

6 medjool dates, pitted

2 teaspoons poppy seeds

1 teaspoon grated lemon zest

Juice of ½ lemon

1 teaspoon vanilla extract

⅛ teaspoon sea salt

In a high-speed blender or a food processor, combine all the ingredients and blend until smooth. Using your hands, form the mixture into 10 balls (each about 1 inch in diameter) and refrigerate until firm, about 30 minutes. Serve chilled. These will stay fresh in an airtight container in the fridge for up to 1 week.

CARB CASH EXCHANGE: 🔲 per bite

CONDIMENTS YOU'LL CRAVE

Don't underestimate the power of a flavorful dip and delicious condiment to transform virtually anything from raw veggies to simply prepared proteins and bowls.

Spicy Avocado Dip

Makes about ¾ cup; serves 3 to 4

A fresh, nutty take on guac, this is perfect for dipping crudités like sliced carrots, cucumber, and bell pepper. It would also be pretty insane (in a good way) on a cauliflower-tortilla taco.

½ avocado, pitted and peeled

¼ cup extra-virgin olive oil

1 lacinato (dinosaur) kale leaf

1 clove garlic

1 shallot

¼ cup salted roasted pistachios

½ serrano chile pepper

Juice of 1 lime

Ground cumin

Blitz all the ingredients up to the lime in a high-speed blender until smooth, then serve topped with cumin to taste. Serve now or store in an airtight container in the fridge for up to 3 days.

CARB CASH EXCHANGE:

Mixed-Olive Tapenade

Makes about ⅓ cup; serves 2 to 3

Yes, you can buy olive tapenade at just about any grocery store these days. But trust me: A store-bought version will pale next to this fresh, vibrant one, which can be used as a dip for crudités, a condiment for wraps, or as a sauce for fish and veggies.

⅓ cup mixed olives, pitted
1 oil-packed anchovy, sliced
1 clove garlic, chopped
2 tablespoons extra-virgin olive oil
½ teaspoon Dijon mustard
1 tablespoon pine nuts

Blitz all the ingredients in a high-speed blender until smooth. Store in an airtight container in the fridge for up to 2 weeks.

CARB CASH EXCHANGE:

SIDES

These sides can be made ahead of time and eaten alone as snacks or paired with protein as part of a lunch or dinner.

Rustic Roasted Mushrooms

Serves 2 to 3

These are ultra-savory and delicious by themselves, or they can multitask in a frittata or as a topping for Cauliflower Pizza Crust (page 139).

- 2 portobello mushrooms, stems and gills removed, cut into ½-inch slices
- 1 leek (white and light green parts), sliced
- ¼ cup olive oil
- Leaves from 1 sprig fresh rosemary
- Leaves from 1 sprig fresh thyme
- Pinch of sea salt

Preheat the oven to 400°F and line a baking sheet with parchment paper. Toss the mushrooms and leek slices with the olive oil, rosemary, thyme, and salt on the prepared baking sheet. Roast for 15 to 20 minutes, flipping once. Serve warm, or save to add to a frittata. Store in an airtight container in the fridge for up to 1 week.

CARB CASH EXCHANGE:

Roasted Sesame-Ginger Brussels Sprouts

Serves 3 to 4

These flavorful, gingery Brussels sprouts are a perfect side dish for virtually any source of protein, or they can be chopped and added to a frittata.

  1 pound Brussels sprouts, trimmed and halved
  2 tablespoons extra-virgin olive oil
  2 tablespoons coconut aminos
  1 clove garlic, minced
  1-inch piece ginger, peeled and grated (about 1 teaspoon)
  Pinch of sea salt
  Pinch of red pepper flakes
  1 tablespoon toasted sesame seeds
  Drizzle of hot toasted sesame oil

Preheat the oven to 400°F and line a baking sheet with parchment paper. In a bowl, toss together the Brussels sprouts, olive oil, coconut aminos, garlic, ginger, salt, and red pepper flakes. Place the sprouts on the prepared baking sheet and pour the remaining oil mixture on top. Roast for 15 to 20 minutes, flipping once, or until golden. Top with sesame seeds and hot toasted sesame oil.

CARB CASH EXCHANGE:

Broiled Sesame Asparagus

Serves 3 to 4

This is such a simple dish and yet it's so, so good! It works incredibly well as a side or a snack; plus, the leftovers can be added to Baked Frittata Muffins (page 156).

    1 pound asparagus, ends trimmed
    3 tablespoons extra-virgin olive oil
    1 tablespoon brown rice vinegar
    1 tablespoon coconut aminos
    1 tablespoon toasted sesame seeds
    Hot sesame oil
    Sea salt and pepper

Preheat the oven to broil and line a baking sheet with parchment paper. In a bowl, combine the asparagus, olive oil, vinegar, and coconut aminos; turn to coat evenly. Place the asparagus on the baking sheet so the stalks are evenly spaced and not touching; pour the remaining oil mixture on top. Broil for 15 minutes, flipping once halfway through. Serve warm, topped with the sesame seeds, hot sesame oil, salt, and pepper to taste.

CARB CASH EXCHANGE:

Cauliflower "Popcorn"

Serves 3 to 4

Something wonderful happens when you roast cauliflower florets with the right flavor combos. I'm not sure why, but the florets start tasting a bit like popcorn. This recipe also works great with turmeric for a flavor (and antioxidant) boost.

    1 head cauliflower, cut into small florets
    ¼ cup extra-virgin olive oil
    ¼ cup apple cider vinegar
    ½ teaspoon garlic powder
    ½ teaspoon onion powder
    Dash of ground cumin
    Pinch of sea salt

Preheat the oven to 425°F and line a baking sheet with parchment paper. In a bowl, combine the cauliflower, olive oil, vinegar, spices, and salt and toss to coat evenly. Place the florets on the prepared baking sheet so they are evenly spaced and not touching; pour the remaining oil mixture on top. Roast for 25 minutes, flipping once, or until golden. Enjoy!

CARB CASH EXCHANGE:

Sweet Potato Curly Fries

Serves 2

Ever since I realized that I could use my spiralizer to make curly fries, life hasn't been the same. Not only are these fries adorable, but the spiralizing process cuts the baking time down by more than half, which is invaluable when you're pressed for time. (For maximum efficiency, I use a spiralizing attachment that works with my standing mixer.)

1 skin-on sweet potato, spiralized on the thickest setting

2 tablespoons-extra virgin olive oil

3 tablespoons apple cider vinegar

½ teaspoon garlic powder

½ teaspoon onion powder

Dash of ground cumin

Pinch of sea salt

Preheat the oven to 400°F and line a baking sheet with parchment paper. In a bowl, combine the sweet potato, olive oil, vinegar, garlic powder, onion powder, cumin, and sea salt and toss to coat evenly. Place in a single layer on the baking sheet, making sure not to over-crowd the fries, and pour the remaining oil mixture on top. Roast the fries for 20 minutes, flipping once halfway through, or until they reach their desired crispiness. (If you don't have a spiralizer and you've cut the fries, you'll need to roast them longer, about 40 minutes.)

CARB CASH EXCHANGE: [○○○] per ½ sweet potato

NOT-TOO-SWEET SWEETS

SIMPLE CHOCOLATE DRIZZLE

Serves 2

When that chocolate craving comes on strong, it's nice to have the good stuff on hand. I love this drizzle on roasted nuts and fresh raspberries.

2 ounces unsweetened baking chocolate (100 percent cacao)
1 tablespoon maple syrup
Pinch of sea salt

In a double boiler or heatproof bowl placed over a pot of simmering water, melt together the chocolate and maple syrup. Stir until the mixture is completely smooth. Season with salt to taste. Remove from the heat and drizzle or dip as desired.

CARB CASH EXCHANGE: [○○○] Make sure to account for the carb cost of the foods you're drizzling this on, as well (such as fruit).

ANDIE AND EVA'S CHOCO-AVO PUDDING

Serves 4

My hometown pal Andie Yamagami also happens to be the owner of San Francisco's clean-food mecca As Quoted. I was lucky enough to have her create an extra simple and insanely flavorful sweet treat specifically for this book, and it does not disappoint. Fun fact: Andie delivered her second child, baby girl Eva, soon after sending me this recipe (how *badass* is that?), hence the name. Feel free to top this with unsweetened shredded coconut or roasted nuts for a mixed-media effect.

2 ripe avocados, pitted, peeled, and cut into chunks
½ cup unsweetened nut milk, such as almond, cashew, or hemp
¼ cup unsweetened raw cacao powder
⅓ cup maple syrup
½ teaspoon vanilla extract
Pinch of sea salt

In a high-speed blender or a food processor, combine all the ingredients and blend until smooth. Separate into 4 containers and refrigerate for at least 2 hours. Store in an airtight container in the fridge for up to 3 days.

CARB CASH EXCHANGE: 🗒️

CASHEW MILK

Makes about 2½ cups

Making nut milk is one of those things that sounds like a big production, but is so far from it. I make this recipe whenever I can because I find that unlike most store-bought nut milks, this one is extra creamy, almost like full-fat cow's milk. Plus, most store-bought alternative milks out there have stabilizers and gums that I'd rather avoid if I can. The vanilla adds just the right amount of sweetness sans actual sugar.

    1 cup raw cashews
    2 cups filtered water
    ¼ teaspoon vanilla extract
    Pinch of sea salt
    ¼ teaspoon ground cinnamon

Put the cashews in a bowl and add cold water to cover by 1 inch. Soak overnight or for at least 8 hours on the countertop. Rinse the cashews and drain them well. Transfer the soaked cashews to a high-speed blender and add the filtered water. Blend until cashews are finely ground. Squeeze the mixture through a nut milk bag or a square of cheesecloth into a bowl or pitcher, discarding solids. Mix in the vanilla extract, salt, and cinnamon. Drink immediately, or cover and store in the fridge for up to 3 days.

CARB CASH EXCHANGE:

THE PUZZLE COMPLETED

If you're feeling a bit overwhelmed, I can hardly blame you. I've thrown a lot of info and recipes at you. But here's the bottom line: Assembling delicious, satisfying, good-for-you meals isn't that big a deal when you set yourself up by pre-prepping your ingredients—especially when you use the formulas provided in this chapter as a guide. Now you have the opportunity to translate your intentions into actions by putting all the pieces together and creating a weekly meal plan. Here's what one might look like with four carb servings per day—if you want to lose weight, for instance. (If you're trying to maintain your weight, you might have *six* carb servings per day, which means you could add in an extra serving of sweet potato, plus a couple of squares of dark chocolate.) No need to follow this to the letter; it's simply meant to be an example to steer you in the right direction.

SAMPLE SEVEN-DAY MEAL PLAN

	Breakfast	Snack	Lunch	Snack	Dinner
MONDAY	Raspberry Bar **1½ CARB SERVINGS**	Brussels Sprouts Chips	Spicy Cabbage Mix with Garlic Crema Dressing and tomatoes or salsa, ½ avocado, and 4 to 6 ounces protein, along with Sweet Potato Curly Fries **1 CARB SERVING**	Orange-Rosemary Pecans **½ CARB SERVING**	Cauliflower Rice, Mexi-Cali Style with Garlic Crema Dressing and 4 to 6 ounces protein Dessert: Simple Chocolate Drizzle on ¼ cup roasted nuts **1 CARB SERVING**
TUESDAY	Baked Frittata Muffins with Simple Pesto Sauce, plus 1 cup raspberries **1 CARB SERVING**	Spicy Avocado Dip with crudités	Spicy Cabbage Mix with Chinese Chicken Salad Dressing, along with ¼ avocado, sliced scallions, toasted sesame seeds, and 4 to 6 ounces protein **1 CARB SERVING**	Chocolate-Orange Energy Bites **2 CARB SERVINGS**	Cauliflower Rice, Bibimbap Style, with 4 to 6 ounces protein
WEDNES-DAY	Super-Simple-Smoothie **2 CARB SERVINGS**	Spicy Mixed Nuts	Cauliflower Tortillas with Spicy Cabbage Mix and Garlic Crema Dressing, along with tomatoes or salsa, ¼ avocado, ⅓ cup quinoa, and 4 to 6 ounces protein **1 CARB SERVING**	Andie and Eva's Choco-Avo Pudding **1 CARB SERVING**	Kelp noodles with Sesame Tahini Sauce, along with toasted sesame seeds and 4 to 6 ounces protein

(continued on next page)

	Breakfast	Snack	Lunch	Snack	Dinner
THURS-DAY	Chia Seed Pudding 1 CARB SERVING	Cashew Milk with ¾ cup blue-berries 1 CARB SERVING	Zoodles with Simple Pesto Sauce and 4 to 6 ounces protein	Half an avo-cado with a pinch of sea salt	Broiled Sesame Asparagus and 4 to 6 ounces protein Dessert: Maple- Sesame Cashews with Simple Choco-late Drizzle 2 CARB SERVINGS
FRIDAY	Cashew Milk with Baked Frittata Muffins	Maple-Sesame Cashews 1 CARB SERVING	Spicy Cabbage Salad with Chinese Chicken Salad Dressing, along with ¼ avocado, sliced scallions, toasted sesame seeds, and 4 to 6 ounces protein	Lemon–Poppy Seed Bites 2 CARB SERVINGS	Zoodles with Curry in a Hurry sauce, along with cashews and 4 to 6 ounces protein 1 CARB SERVING
SATUR-DAY	Baked Frit-tata Muf-fins with Lemon-Poppy Seed Bites 2 CARB SERVINGS	Mixed Olive Tapenade with crudités	Roasted Sesame Ginger Brussels Sprouts, along with ⅓ cup quinoa and 4 to 6 ounces protein 1 CARB SERVING	Cauliflower "Popcorn"	Zoodles with Epic Vegetable Bolognese and 4 to 6 ounces protein, plus Sweet Potato Curly Fries 1 CARB SERVING
SUNDAY	"Buttermilk" Pancakes with ghee or unsweet-ened nut butter topped with cinnamon 2 CARB SERVINGS	Cashew Milk	Spicy Cabbage Mix with Spicy Thai dressing, toasted cashews, sliced scallions, and toasted sesame seeds, along with 4 to 6 ounces protein	Spicy Avo-cado Dip with crudités	Rustic Roasted Mushrooms with Brussels Sprouts Chips, along with ⅔ cup quinoa and 4 to 6 ounces protein 2 CARB SERVINGS

As you've probably noticed, this approach picks up where a lot of plans leave off—namely, in real life. Thanks to its built-in flexibility, you can make sure this carb-savvy, modified-Paleo style of eating works for *you* and your lifestyle. When you pre-prep ingredients, you're precommitting to eating healthfully throughout the week, so you can save your willpower for times when you really need it. In the meantime, the strategies outlined in this chapter will help take the guesswork out of what to actually eat every day. In the process, you'll be resetting your hormones and reclaiming your ability to listen to your body's hunger and satiety cues. Not only will you be doing your future self a major favor, but you'll also reap more immediate benefits as you start feeling more balanced (and less chaotic). Along the way, you'll naturally enhance your relationship with food, making it more flexible and satisfying.

8

Keep the Magic Alive

Truth be told, things can get stale in the dining room, just as they can in the bedroom. Routines are pretty clutch for modern life, especially in terms of workouts, sleep, and childrearing—but when it comes to passion in relationships, copy-and-paste predictability can really kill the mood. It's just not all that stimulating when you know *exactly* what's coming next, play by play. But that's kind of the default natural progression in relationships, isn't it? At first it's all excitement and fireworks, and then we tend to settle in; we get ultra-comfortable and preoccupied with other stuff, and ultimately stop putting in the effort needed to keep things fresh. Well, there's certainly a food-relationship equivalent to wearing granny panties and having exclusively lights-out missionary, and it's eating the same thing day after day, thinking of food as simply "fuel," and not putting much thought into making things flavorful. The point is: Passion ruts happen—in our food lives and our romantic ones—and the key to getting things back on a more tantalizing track is to break the spell of perpetual sameness.

I speak from extensive personal experience on this front because I'm a serious creature of habit and have burned out many former favorite foods from sheer overuse. The issue: Even if what you're eating is delicious, if it's the same thing you ate yesterday and the day before that—without much variation—it's going to stop doing the satisfaction trick. That's because perpetual food ruts don't just bore our taste buds; they can also encourage us to zone out while eating, kind of like putting ourselves on attention cruise control. Researchers refer to this phenomenon—mentally disengaging when we're exposed to the same old stuff—as *neural priming*. It more or less means that when we're first introduced to something new (like a seasonal Sweetgreen salad), parts of our brain (including the beloved PFC) perk up and are like "Oh, hi! Who are *you*?!" In other words, we tune in and take notice. *Neural priming* kicks in once we've had that same salad over and over on a repetitive loop, and instead of perking up, those once eager and active brain regions are like "BRB. Let yourself in."

In fact, the PFC is especially sensitive to repetition and novelty, and there is pretty cool research involving brain scans to prove it. A scientific paper in the March 2003 issue of *Nature Reviews Neuroscience* revealed what anyone who has been bored to oblivion by a painfully dry textbook or monotone lecture has experienced: The brain responds to repetitive stimuli with less neural activity, but responds to comparatively novel stimuli with more activity and attention.

This natural tendency can (and often does) work in our favor, especially when it comes to adopting skills that eventually don't require too much brainpower or undivided concentration. But when it comes to *actually eating*, we want to be attuned in real time because attention paid to what we're eating while we're eating plays a major role in helping us feel satisfied afterward. Plain and simple: If we want to continue making conscious food choices with the PFC engaged (and continue feeling satisfied by the foods we choose), it's wise to avoid boring it into submission. The way to do that is to make a point of building in a hint of newness whenever possible.

After all, it's easy to get stuck in your comfort zone where you cling to the same old, same old foods, preparation styles, and taste sensations—and that's because they're familiar and that feels good. But when familiarity segues into serious food monotony, it can set you up to stray from your good intentions. Just like boredom in your romantic relationship can give you a wandering eye, the same thing can happen with your eating habits. Neither scenario means the relationship is doomed, but it *is* a sign that something's missing. With respect to your food relationship, there's no need to do a complete 180, *Eat, Pray, Love* style; instead, just take some proactive steps to spice up the relationship you have. I'm not talking about ditching your previous routine—routines are good. This is really about keeping your meals engaging and satisfying and avoiding chronic food-rut territory. Yes, keeping the spark alive takes work— but not as much as you may think. Here are some totally doable strategies to help keep your food life fresh.

LET THE SEASONS GUIDE YOU

It's easy to get overwhelmed by all the recipes and meal possibilities out there (hello, decision fatigue), so narrowing the field and bypassing the "what to eat?" conundrum is key. A great way to do this is by going to your local farmers' market and letting the seasonal options guide your meal-prep plans. Plus, if you're selecting produce that's in season at its natural peak, you'll be getting the best flavor. So stock up on Brussels sprouts and root vegetables (like parsnips and rutabagas) in the fall; cabbage and broccoli rabe in the winter; artichokes, asparagus, and ramps in the spring; and summer squash, tomatoes, and cucumbers in the summer. If you spot an item you've never seen or prepared before (like sunchokes or fiddlehead ferns), ask the vendors how they recommend preparing it (they usually have the best insider tips). Also, check out hybrid veggies—like broccoflower (broccoli cross-pollinated with cauliflower), kalettes (Brussels sprouts crossed with kale), and broccolini (a mash-up of standard broccoli and Chinese broccoli)—which combine the sensory and nutritional characteristics of two different plants.

TWEAK THE FLAVORS

No need to reinvent the wheel. Breaking out of a food rut can be as simple as a few choice flavor tweaks. You can do this by switching up the vinegar in your salad dressings; for instance, if you tend to stick with white wine vinegar, try experimenting with apple cider, red wine, or Champagne vinegars. Same thing with oils. Olive oil is incredible and oh-so-versatile, but different healthy oils like sesame, walnut, and avocado can add a whole new flavor dimension that you didn't see coming. Adding citrus zest to salads, bowls, fish, or chicken is another easy way to brighten up otherwise familiar foods.

Don't be afraid to think outside the box and experiment. Getting tired of Andie and Eva's Choco-Avo Pudding (page 174)? Throw some chili powder or peppermint extract in there—and *boom*—brand spanking new. If you know your go-to supermarket like the back of your hand, it's easy to get into the routine of buying the same old stuff. So shake things up by checking out ethnic food markets—Japanese, Persian, Indian, Mexican, and so on—to broaden your repertoire of tasty ingredients.

PLAY WITH THE PREP

How you prepare certain foods can really change up the flavor. Don't feel like eating crudités? Try blanching veggies instead (it varies the taste and the texture a bit). Bored with your usual poached or rotisserie chicken? Try braising, which seriously amps up the flavor. You can also go off-road by mastering a favorite recipe and then modifying it. Love the Raspberry Bars (page 157) so much that you could make them with your eyes closed? Now try them with blueberries and orange zest instead. Amazing. While pesto zoodles and cauliflower-crust pizza taste incredible topped with raw cherry tomatoes, roasted cherry tomatoes with balsamic vinegar can provide a different and moodier flavor vibe. Similarly, lightly charring sliced citrus fruits (like lemon, orange, and lime) brings out the natural sweetness while toning down the acidity, which can be a great way to add new depth to vinaigrettes, dips, and proteins like grilled fish or roasted chicken. Taking a cooking class every so often can also really help get the creative juices flowing.

ADD UMAMI

One of my recipe-testing mantras is: When in doubt, add umami, which is often referred to as the fifth basic taste (alongside sweet, sour, salty, and bitter). The Japanese word, which is fairly buzzy these days, describes the earthy, savory flavors often associated with cooked meat, aged cheeses, mushrooms, soy sauce, and miso. The flavor actually comes from a naturally occurring amino acid called glutamate, which amps up flavor in food. The more glutamate a particular food or dish has, the more flavorful it is, which is why traditional Japanese stocks (dashi) almost always start with kombu: dried seaweed that's loaded with glutamate. In the West, it's more common to use not-so-healthy forms of glutamate (like MSG, or monosodium glutamate) to enhance flavor. But luckily for us, there are tons of widely available and healthy sources of umami, particularly mushrooms and fermented foods (like sauerkraut, kimchi, fish sauce, and coconut aminos), which is why these pop up so frequently in my recipes. Plus, research suggests that adding umami to a dish can enhance satisfaction as well as flavor.

EXPERIMENT WITH MIXED MEDIA

Think about a delicious bowl of guacamole: the smooth, creamy chunks of avocado, the juicy diced tomato, the sharp, fiery pop of chopped onions and chiles. Now imagine you took all those ingredients and pulsed them in a blender until the consistency resembled a thick smoothie. Not as appetizing, right? In theory, it's all the same ingredients and flavors, so what's the problem? Well, for starters, that sounds like a meal for a toddler. Plus, when it comes to food, sensory excitement doesn't just include taste; it includes textures, too. The fact is, one-note foods without any real textural variation aren't that exciting—for our taste buds or our brains. There's actually a full-blown scientific term for this—*dynamic contrast*—which essentially means that when foods that are eaten together have sensory attributes that differ from one another, it makes for a more appealing, titillating, and attention-grabbing experience. I'm not suggesting you go full molecular gastronomy with ridiculous foams and liquid nitrogen and whatnot, but I do recommend adding in some mixed media when possible to help excite your senses.

By playing with texture, you can make a familiar dish feel shiny and new. So you might pair something crunchy with something ultra-smooth, like topping chocolate-avocado pudding with toasted coconut flakes, or adding sesame seeds or toasted pistachios to creamy dips. Similarly, you can combine something juicy and astringent with a more delicate food (like adding a handful of pomegranate seeds to roasted eggplant) and double the thrill for your senses.

PAIR SURPRISING INGREDIENTS

Just like some people are pretty much meant to be pairs (Goldie and Kurt, Oprah and Gayle), some flavor combos are so obvious they feel like they should be sold together, like tomato and basil. Other times, there are pairings that seem a little less obvious but are somehow oh-so-compatible. Whether it's because they're synergistic or complementary, or they manage to bring out the best in each other, interesting flavor combos can add a welcome dose of wow-factor newness to your food world. Here are a few of my favorites that will hopefully spark some pairing ideas that speak to you:

Kabocha squash + colatura: When I was living in New York I burned out on kabocha squash pretty hard, thanks to very frequent visits to one of my favorite restaurants in the West Village. I loved that kabocha squash so much and had it so often that I kind of maxed out and stopped ordering it for *years*. But recently I spotted a particularly good-looking one at a restaurant in LA so I ordered it, and let me tell you: It wasn't just ridiculously good; it was *different*, with a depth of flavor I hadn't experienced before. When I asked the server, she let me in on the secret: colatura. I spent the car ride home Googling this mystical ingredient, which is made from the juice of fermented anchovies; it has since become a staple in my arsenal of flavors. Trust me on this one.

Kimchi + roasted nut butter: Full disclosure: I'd eat kimchi straight out of the jar, I love it that much. But something really amazing happens when it's paired with roasted nut butter (almond butter, cashew butter, you name it). A couple of years ago, I discovered this combo from an expert fermenter during a workshop: When she mentioned it, everyone in the room looked at her like she was absolutely bananas, but she maintained such a confident *just wait, you'll see* smirk that I had to take the challenge. *OMG.* That woman is a complete flavor genius. The nut butter tempered the fierce acidity of the pungent, vinegary kimchi in all the right ways and added a little something extra I never knew I needed. I'm assuming this would work with roasted nuts, too. If you're a kimchi lover, get involved.

Sauerkraut + avocado: They say opposites attract and these two foods couldn't be more different, but they are kind of the perfect pair. Somewhere between the delicate, buttery avo and the sharp, garlicky kraut, serious flavor magic happens. Half an avocado topped with extra-sour sauerkraut is one of my all-time favorite snacks.

Chocolate + cardamom: The whole chocolate/chili thing is definitely delish, but it's also nothing new. If you're into a spicy, chocolaty flavor combo, consider pairing dark chocolate or Simple Chocolate Drizzle (page 173) with cardamom for a more complex, warm, almost citrusy vibe.

The Flavor Wheel

Now that you have a window into my taste-bud soul, it's time for you to discover pairings that speak to *your* flavor palette. Check out the flavor wheel on the next page—which illustrates contrasting and complementary taste sensations—and then get creative by combining two or three different flavors that *you* think would go well together. For example, if your go-to snack is typically roasted nuts and a piece of fruit, consider experimenting with a sweet-umami-salty snack combo such as goji berries, nori strips (or furikake), and salted roasted nuts. If your favorite salad isn't exciting you the way it used to, think about punching it up with a sour-spicy-umami dressing with Dijon mustard, grated ginger, and a splash of coconut aminos, along with chopped radicchio or shredded Brussels sprouts (bitter). Really, the combos are endless, which comes in especially handy when meals are starting to feel a little *too* predictable.

Sure, every once in a while you may make an epic flavor fail (like that one time I mixed roasted nuts with wasabi, coconut aminos, and coconut oil, and it was one of the worst things I have ever tasted, like *ever*). But you really won't know unless you experiment.

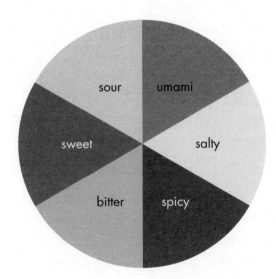

Examples from the Food Therapist Plan
Sweet
maple syrup
dates
dried mulberries
vanilla extract
pomegranate seeds

Umami
coconut aminos

nori/furikake
fish sauce/colatura
mushrooms
caramelized onions

Salty
olives
anchovies
capers
pickled veggies
pepperoncini

Spicy
ginger
garlic
basil
chiles
cinnamon
cloves
cumin

Bitter
very dark chocolate
coffee
horseradish
radishes
cilantro

cabbage/Brussels sprouts
arugula/radicchio

Sour
lemon/lime
grapefruit
mustard
sauerkraut/kimchi
vinegar (apple cider, balsamic, white wine, brown rice, etc.)
coconut milk kefir/coconut water kefir
kombucha

Keep It Colorful

There's nothing quite like an attractive plate of vibrant, color-ful food to excite the senses. You don't have to channel Andy Warhol and make your food look like pop art, but when possible, use color to liven things up: Instead of going with the usual white cauliflower, try yellow; swap regular sweet potatoes for purple ones; or choose rainbow-hued carrots instead of the standard orange.

I once saw a woman working at a clothing store wearing a dress that was the same as one I owned, but somehow hers looked different and more appealing. There was a period when I used to wear that dress *all the time*, but eventually I grew bored with it, and it was banished to wardrobe purgatory at the back of my closet. Then I realized she was wearing hers backward! (Or, was *mine* backward?) Either way, she had totally flipped the script on our dress. When I got home I tried mine on her way, and it was like the dress was legitimately new again. Think of the advice in this chapter as the food version of tweaking an outfit you already own in order to keep your healthy-eating repertoire enjoyable and non-yawn-worthy.

When it comes down to it, I'm a firm believer that food is nourishment but also a substantial source of pleasure. And it really deserves to be both. After all, the ultimate goal isn't just to make more conscious healthy food decisions, but also to thoroughly *enjoy* eating. Plus, having both elements is seriously crucial to making this whole thing work for the long haul. The reality is, healthy relationships are not simply first dates and honeymoon sex; they're also about coordinating schedules, making compromises, and divvying up duties. Which is why it's so important to make an effort to keep the day-to-day stuff fun and fresh, too.

9

Get the %&^# Out of Your Own Way

Even in the best relationships, sh*t happens and you have to forgive your partner (within reason) or apologize for your own mistakes so you can both move on. Let's be real: Taking that high road isn't always easy, but the alternative—perpetual passive-aggressiveness, tension, and Arctic-chill distance—is much less desirable. The same is true of your relationship with food. The difference is that while we tend to forgive our loved ones for being imperfect human beings who don't always behave the way we'd like them to, we don't often do ourselves the same solid, *especially* when it comes to eating. When we deviate from our intended food plans, instead of acknowledging our supreme disappointment and then dropping it, we tend to go full disgruntled Walter White—with thoughts like, *"You #$%^ed it all up!! Ugh, you're pathetic. Of course, this is what* *happened; this is what always happens. You're literally the worst."* But as we know from the *what-the-hell effect*, that hostile approach doesn't just feel like crap; it backfires by making it virtually impossible to move forward. Instead, we're thrown into the shame cycle, where we get stuck. Note to self: This can also happen when you feel like you've hit a weight-loss plateau or when you compare your progress or efforts to what other people are doing. Playing the comparison game pretty much always makes you feel like garbage.

I know, because I've been there. Let me start by saying that I am no Gigi Hadid, and I definitely have not-thrilled-with-my-body days, but more often than not I feel pretty decent naked. That is, unless I shower with a supermodel. When I moved back to LA from NYC, my bathroom was being renovated, so I showered at the gym on a regular basis. That was fine until the moment I walked out of the shower at the exact same time as a supermodel and we were both facing a wall of mirrors. Just to be clear: I don't mean someone who's so attractive that she *could* be a supermodel; I'm talking about an actual, legit supermodel (who will remain unnamed). So there we were, my naked body and her supermodel naked body, side by side, and even though I had just worked out and had been feeling pretty good, when I compared my bod to this beautiful woman's bod I felt, well, not so great. I honestly had to hit my mental pause button and remind myself that not only is this woman a supermodel, but also her beauty doesn't make mine any less real. We're just different people with different bodies. Truth be told, if that situation ever presents itself again, I'll probably need to give myself the same pep talk. But the point is, we're all going to be tempted to make those unrealistic comparisons now and then, but they really don't do us any favors.

By now you've had a chance to get intimately acquainted with your personal eating-related obstacles and find ways to sidestep them to a certain extent. All the skills you've honed so far—tuning in to yourself while eating, connecting with your future self, planning ahead, keeping the PFC engaged, and so on—will undoubtedly set you up to make consciously healthy food choices more regularly. But I'd be doing you a major disservice by leaving it there, because doing the afore-mentioned work won't make you immune to future glitches and setbacks. Roadblocks will still pop up, and the better you are at spotting them on the horizon and not letting them break your spirit, the more swiftly you can move past them. The key is to find ways to recapture momentum and get back on track when your progress stagnates or your best-laid plans go off script, because at some point they most certainly will.

I didn't mean for that to sound dark, just realistic. After all, when you're under loads of stress or you're getting your butt kicked by a major life transition (even an exciting one like graduating, getting a new job, or moving in with your S.O.), your good intentions can get lost in the shuffle. The same is true when the holidays, a trip, or houseguests distract you from your intended food game. As you know by now, you're a lot more vulnerable to making hasty food choices with the PFC off duty, when your thoughts are consumed with other stuff. Detours can also happen when something that *was* motivating you (a wedding, a beach vacation, or some other event) has passed. Under these circumstances, it's easy to feel like you've backpedaled and your progress is ruined (there goes that black-and-white thinking again). In these low moments, we're quick to call ourselves out for not having willpower, but oftentimes that's not the case at all. More often it has a lot to do with the faulty mindsets and wonky logic—particularly, moral licensing and loopholes—we use to rationalize ditching our long-term goals to serve our right-now wants.

Moral licensing is the idea that "good" behavior offsets or legitimizes "bad" behavior. It's a way of justifying pouncing on a right-now desire by referencing past or current ethical behavior. The basis is completely understandable: In general, people like to feel and be seen as being "good" and doing the "right" thing. But we're often swayed to behave in ways that might call our "goodness" into question. For instance, when a coworker asks for a ride to the airport or a friend asks for a donation for her kid's school function, you might find yourself with a dilemma: You don't really want to do it, but at the same time you don't want to feel like or be thought of as a lousy person. In these tricky situations, it's common to use moral licensing as a way to let yourself off the hook. It's kind of like ethical accounting—doing a quick rundown in your head of examples that point to you being a stand-up person or a good friend—which can empower you to be like, "Love you, but can't help you out this time." Well, we do the same thing with food. You may even be intimately familiar with this line of thinking: "I've been *so* good lately, I really deserve this giant plate of pasta."

Or, "I've had the most brutal week, so I've seriously earned this pastry." And also, "I'm *so* much better than I used to be; this gorge sesh really isn't *that* bad."

But when it comes to eating, the big issue with employing moral licensing has little to do with the indulgence itself; it's the fallacy that deciding whether or not to indulge is a matter of vice or virtue. It's not. Unlike, say, debating whether to cheat on your partner (or your taxes), deciding what to eat vs. what *not* to eat isn't a moral dilemma. Let's be clear about this: Making consciously healthy food choices is great and I highly recommend it, but choosing a less-healthy track isn't somehow *less ethical*. But when we apply shady logic like this, we bypass a really important step: weighing our right-now wants against our future-self desires. This carries us further away from our get-healthy goals without us even realizing it, and then we end up attributing that intention-action gap to lacking willpower and resolve. That's not the case, but viewing it this way can lead you to throw your hands up in frustration—or worse, sink into over-it apathy.

The other problem with this mentality is the assumption that you need an external excuse or extenuating circumstance to indulge. You don't. If you want the croissant or pizza or dough-nut or fries…go for it and enjoy the *$%^&* out of it. I mean it: *Every. Single. Bite.* It really doesn't matter if you've attained inbox zero or you've had the worst week of your life. You're welcome to indulge, regardless of those backdrops—as long as you do so consciously and take responsibility for the decision.

Similar to moral licensing, loopholes are another common way we use flawed logic to explain why we should be excused from sticking with a healthy habit. *"This doesn't count," "It's the weekend," "It's summer,"* or *"I'm on vacation"*—you name it; it's probably been used as a rationalization for why it's cool for someone to ditch the plan and act in the moment. Again, the issue isn't the desire to let loose; in fact, *please* do let loose here and there, *especially* on vacation or when it's important to you. But pretending that certain days and seasons count less than others do isn't part of the deal, because when you indulge under that misleading pretense, there's a really good chance you'll feel discouraged and at a loss when you get to the other side. There are no hall passes, and that's because you don't need a hall pass when it comes to eating. *End of story.* So the next time you're faced with a tricky food decision, stop asking yourself "How good have I been?" or "How much do I deserve this?" or "What day is it?" Instead, hit the pause button and consider, "How much do I *want* this particular food?" and let your answer guide your behavior.

THE (INADVERTENT) SELF-SABOTAGE SURVIVAL GUIDE

At the risk of sounding like a broken record, let me say it again: The goal isn't to make sure you never veer off your desired eating path; it's to forgive yourself for taking a step back so you can take another step forward. Sure, feeling like you've backpedaled after all your hard work is especially frustrating, but hey, it happens. *Seriously.* So cut your losses: Forgive yourself, so you can move the #$%^ on. By redirecting your disappoint-ment with self-compassion, you can skip the paralyzing shame cycle and get back into a rational frame of mind.

To do this, it helps to start by taking a critical but drama-free look at why you went astray. After all, it's just not realistic to think you won't make some impulsive food choices along the way. Rather than playing the shame game, it's far more productive to try to understand the nature of those deci-sions (specifically, how, when, and why you lost self-control) so you can figure out how to deal more effectively in the future. Psychologists call this *cognitive reframing*, which really just means identifying counterproductive thoughts, disputing them, and then replacing them with more constructive ones. Regardless of the obstacles you typically struggle with, here are some examples of how this process might play out:

Your first thought is: I *really* shouldn't have eaten that.

Your second thought is: *Well, you know what?*—it was deli-cious and I enjoyed every morsel. The best thing I can do now is avoid diving headfirst into shame city.

Your first thought is: I'm just not good at eating healthfully.

Your second thought is: *Hold up.* I've been putting so much more thought into my food choices than I used to. It's still not easy, and there's definitely room for improvement, but I'm getting better at this.

Your first thought is: Ugh, why did I have to mess up my progress like that?!

Your second thought is: Honestly, I may have been getting a little too rigid; now I know that I've got to give myself more wiggle room so I don't get the urge to straight-up revolt.

The point is, when you approach diet detours rationally and compassionately, rather than spinning your wheels with self-inflicted shame, you can focus your energy on turning all that valuable self-knowledge into a useful road map for the future. Once you understand which specific situations and factors make you vulnerable to noshing impulsively, you can plan for them in advance. I'm talking about an if/then game plan (aka an *implementation intention*, a fancy phrase for an effective self-regulatory strategy) that lets you map out your approach to handling potential roadblocks that tend to trip you up. The basic idea is to come up with tactics for "If this happens (no biggie), then I'll do this" scenarios—it's like having a designated Plan B for when things go amiss, so the detour doesn't stop you in your tracks. For example, if you found it challenging to eat healthfully during the holidays this year, you could decide to give yourself a bit more wiggle room next year, while still doing your best to make conscious food choices; and *if* you find yourself feeling not-so-balanced come January, *then* you might plan to go back to Phase I for a week or two to reboot. No guilt, no questions asked. That's your *if/then* game plan. Ironically, having it in place ahead of time takes some serious pressure off self-control, which can actually help you better regulate your behavior. In fact, research in the *Journal of Experimental Social Psychology* found that when people experienced ego depletion during a perplexing mental task, forming implementation intentions helped them improve their performance on a subsequent (equally frustrating) task. The same perks can occur when you prepare for potential eating-related obstacles in advance. It's almost like once you accept and acknowledge that you won't always self-regulate perfectly and you have a plan for how to deal if you deviate from your intended food plan, there's less pressure on you to exercise perfect self-control, which helps it come more naturally.

You can start personalizing your *if/then* approach, based on your food-related obstacles. Here are some examples, based on common setbacks that occur with each type of food-related hang-up:

Trust Issues

You reverted back to old habits at a family-style dinner or buffet—and overate big time.

First, recognize that this type of free-for-all dining setup is challenging for everyone. Then, get strategic for next time: Before loading up your plate, take a beat to survey all your options, then choose ones that are in sync with your good intentions and appeal to you the most. If you were shopping for jeans, you probably wouldn't buy the first pair in sight; instead, you'd peruse and try on various options before committing. Same goes for food.

The Pleaser Trap

At a dinner with friends, you caved to pressure and ended up eating what they ordered instead of sticking to your own preferences.

Acknowledge that social pressure can be hard to resist. Then, come up with a game plan and a miniscript for what you could do differently next time. Check out the menu beforehand and order first, if possible. Also, it can help to preempt any expectations from your dining companions, with a comment like, "It sounds like you're interested in a shared-plates type of thing... but I'm going to fly solo today." The message is friendly but firm, making it clear that this issue is not up for debate.

Fear of the Mundane

You celebrated a major work victory carb-coma style; now, you're feeling bad about ditching your good intentions.

For starters, congrats on crushing it; you definitely deserve to reward yourself for your hard work. But since your natural inclination is to self-treat with food, precommit to choosing an inedible yet still feel-good payoff. The next time you're coming up on a productivity benchmark, closing a major deal, or due for another celebration, plan on meeting some of your favorite people someplace enjoyable and memorable like a spa or a concert. You can still go out to dinner, but this way, the meal isn't the sole celebratory activity so you're less likely to use the occasion as a license to lose control.

A Craving for Control

You ate some "bad" foods last night, and now you can't stop beating yourself up for it.

Hopefully, you enjoyed yourself in the moment, but either way, it's time to move on. For starters, one of the reasons this plan works so well is because it builds in stuff like dessert. Dessert isn't something you necessarily need to have every day, but I honestly think it's healthy to make sure your diet isn't purely about nourishment; it should incorporate pleasure, too. If you really went rogue and ended up eating things you didn't intend to, make a mental note of what you could eat instead next time you're craving something sweet (like dark chocolate or cashew cream with berries) or salty (like sweet potato chips and guac). Building in *conscious* indulgences can make them less emotionally loaded and thus less likely to trip you up.

A Hot-and-Cold Pattern

Some friends have become big believers in the new _____ diet, and before you've had a chance to think it through, you've joined them.

You're a newness enthusiast, meaning you may always be at least mildly tempted to ditch your current plan for the latest diet trend on the block. Don't sweat it; instead, think about how to get ahead of that inclination by weaving newness into *this* plan to keep it fresh and appealing. (It's an important step for everyone, but especially for you novelty-seekers.) If you catch yourself with a wandering eye, make a commitment to infuse your meals with new flavor and texture combos on the regular; maybe even make a vow to experiment with at least one new preparation style every month.

A Dependence Issue

The stress from a massive work project has sent you snacking around the clock—and now you don't know how to stop.

First, cut yourself some slack and acknowledge that you're bathing in cortisol. Given your history of using food as a crutch for your feelings, stressful periods are always going to be vulnerable zones for you when it comes to noshing. That's why it's important to plan ahead for those times by having alternate coping strategies at the ready. Keep stuff like a foam roller, a soothing essential oil, and a go-to playlist full of chill music by your desk. The next time you're tempted to lunge for a stress-relieving snack, throw on a couple of your favorite songs and roll out or zone out for 5 to 10 minutes.

Put these elements—self-compassion, cognitive reframing, and implementation intentions—together and you'll be well on your way to making this thing work for the long haul (even when things don't go as planned). Look, I know: Changing old habits is hard, and it can take a considerable amount of time for new attitudes and behaviors to become ingrained as your new normal. There will be times when it's easier to stick with the plan—and times when it's not. That's natural. When you feel you're especially at risk for going off course, reacquaint yourself with what you want for your future self and recommit to reaping that payoff down the road. It's also wise to make sure that what was originally motivating you to develop a healthier relationship with food is *still* motivating you; if not, look for new personally meaningful reasons to continue the pursuit and find ways to persuade yourself that you're worth the effort.

As you continue evolving into your future self, do your best to stay honest with yourself about what factors might be holding you back or impeding your progress—whether it's a fear of failure, a sense of unworthiness, faulty thinking, the way you handle stress, or something else. Also, be prepared for the possibility that as your efforts begin to pay off, you may feel a bit... unsettled. Over the years, I've had clients who self-sabotaged their progress to varying degrees, and it wasn't immediately clear to me why they did this. But I've landed on a theory that checks out again and again, and it's something that nobody really talks about, because it's a little taboo: Sometimes it's a bit terrifying to get what you want. For many people who've had their eye on achieving a certain healthy-body goal, they think about it often. The purposeful effort that's employed while working toward that particular goal becomes a comforting, organizing principle in their lives. Without it, they feel adrift.

Plus, in our society, taking steps to improve your health is perceived as a very noble pursuit, and it can feel really freaking good to achieve that. But *then what*? The barrier to dealing with other stuff in your life kind of disappears. It's a bit like the conundrum commitment-phobic serial daters face when they suddenly meet someone really special—it's incredible, but equally alarming because they aren't really prepared for the relationship to actually work. The same thing can happen when people inadvertently sabotage their healthy-eating progress: When you're continuously working toward a get-healthy goal, it can take the pressure off of focusing on the other stuff that needs tending to in your life. It's not that people don't actually want to accomplish that goal, but once they do, they might have to think about what's next in their self-improvement queue. That can feel unnerving and overwhelming. I think part of this stems from the whole "You can't have it all" dialogue that's prevalent in our culture, with the unwritten message being that if we manage to get what we really want, we'll lose something else that's important along the way. But in this case, maybe you do get to have it all—if having it all means not having to choose between digging your body and enjoying food.

Forget the Fairy Tale; Create Your Own Happy Ending

In any successful relationship, there are essential, enduring qualities that go into making it work: Being attentive, empathetic, flexible, communicative, creative, trusting, and self-aware are definite biggies. The same is true for having a healthy connection with food, and it's a conscious choice to approach your relationship this way for the long haul. If you've been putting the strategies from this book into play, you're already developing the self-knowledge and the tools it takes to achieve your get-healthier goals. At this point, the challenge is to own the changes you've made so far and to continue fine-tuning and personalizing the fundamental concepts so they keep working for you. This way, you'll be in a position to direct your good intentions toward your big-picture get-healthy goals, even when you're tired, hangry, heartbroken, or generally *over* being an adult. With that in mind, here are the food-relationship maxims you'll want to keep honoring so you can close your personal intention-action gap and seal the deal.

Be a flirt. If we talked to our crushes the way we talk to ourselves, we'd never make it out of Tinder-text purgatory. Self-compassion is infinitely more motivating than self-criticism. Besides, self-acceptance and a desire for change are not mutually exclusive; you can love and accept yourself *and* still want to improve yourself at the same time. But this means you have to ditch the heckling and join your own team. If you actively tell yourself that you'll never have self-control with food, never stop overeating, or never lose weight, you probably won't do any of those things. On the other hand, if you convince yourself that you have the ability, and that it's just about applying different techniques and strategies, you'll boost the chances that these goals will come to fruition.

Listen up. As any relationship expert will tell you, it's all about communication: Having on-point listening skills is one of the keys to making healthy relationships thrive and last. Our relationship with food and our bodies is no different. Being fully present and engaged allows you to understand what's going on beneath the surface, helping you distinguish between legit physiological hunger and simply having the munchies, or between feeling satisfied and overly stuffed. Tuning in to yourself also helps you respond to fleeting temptations in a cool, calm, and discerning way. Whether you ultimately decide to indulge (or not), really listening to your body enables you to make conscious food choices. So keep listening to those subtle internal hunger and fullness cues that we're so used to ignoring—and trust them to guide you in the right direction.

Keep taking it S-L-O-W. How amazing does it feel when all of your senses are engaged in romantic scenarios, when you're totally in the moment and relishing every detail? You want to do the same thing with your food: savoring every flavor and sensory quality, including taste, smell, touch, sight, and sound. Slowing down and focusing on moment-to-moment experiences with food improves your ability to self-regulate, meaning you're less likely to eat impulsively or with reckless abandonment. So make a concerted effort to fully experience every bite. Put your fork down between bites or switch hands if it helps you honor the speed limit and eat more deliberately.

Combat decision fatigue. Take steps to conserve your willpower by limiting the number of food-related decisions you need to make throughout the day. To provide yourself with the right structure, clean out your fridge and pantry, ditch foods you don't want to be eating, and replace them with better-for-you options. Plan certain meals and prep staple ingredients ahead of time when possible. Peruse menus in advance and precommit to what you'll order when dining out. This way you can save your self-control for when you *really* need it—because there will be times when you will.

Keep in touch with your future self. All too often we accept the casual hookup even when we're ready to settle down, because we can't actually imagine ourselves finding the love of our lives. Research suggests that the less actively we think about our future selves, the more likely we are to say %^&* *it* to our long-term goals. So continue picturing your future self reaping the benefits of a healthy relationship with food and just how good that feels. Remember: *The more detail, the better.* You may even want to drop your future self an e-mail now and then, with anecdotes about your current status and thoughts about your future hopes. It's one of the best ways to close the gap between your intentions and your day-to-day actions.

Learn from the past and the present, then leave it behind. Doomed romantic relationships can teach us a lot about what we want, what we need, what we're willing to tolerate (and what we're not). The same goes for our relationship with food. So whenever your good intentions don't go according to plan, figure out what triggered you to make choices that aren't in line with what you really want. Then drop it. In order to ditch a habit like emotional overeating, you'll want to continue discovering the types of circumstances that often segue into emotional overeating for you. When you do this, it's easier to notice patterns (like when you crave sweets) and when you tend to throw dietary caution to the wind. As self-awareness increases, you'll get better at making conscious food choices; that said, you certainly won't be immune to future obstacles. So continue keeping a watchful eye on the factors that lead you astray, sans cynical snark. Instead, take a close but drama-free look at why you went off course. Learn what you can from the situation, file it under your "personal history," and forge ahead.

Get out of your own way. When you veer off course from your eating intentions, adopt the mantra *Apologize. Mean it. Move on.* (Practice it regularly.) No matter who you are or how far you've come in maintaining your wellness goals, at some point you'll inevitably take a step backward. It can be incredibly frustrating, but it's a normal part of life. To prevent a lapse from derailing your entire mission, do yourself a favor and get out of your own way: Ditch the negative, counterproductive BS and come up with an if/then game plan for how to deal going forward. Keep your eyes focused on your vision for your future self and continue taking one thoughtful step after another to get there.

Keep things fresh. When it comes to your relationship with food, perpetual sameness is one surefire way to make things feel meh; it can also encourage you to stray from your eating intentions. Of course, there will be times when you're in a rush and you just need to eat, but try to make an effort to keep humdrum repetition at bay. Dodge food ruts by making small sensory tweaks to your go-to meals, like adding different vinegars, citrus zests, herbs and spices, or umami to change up the flavor. The point is, do what you can to keep the food magic alive.

Be emotionally available (for what you want). When you're not quite emotionally available for a healthy, grown-up romantic relationship, meeting the person of your dreams can be low-key terrifying. The same thing can happen with get-healthy goals—that is, if you're not actually prepared to reach them. The reality is, when you start breaking down your emotional hang-ups around food, achieving your goals by closing the gap between your get-healthy intentions and your day-to-day actions becomes a lot easier. On one hand, it can be scary to get what you want because then you're unencumbered to live your life and start accomplishing all the stuff you've been putting off. But it can also be incredibly gratifying if you let yourself own the win and all the mixed feelings that come with it. You deserve the good stuff in life, and feeling comfortable in your own skin is a major part of that.

Look, we're all human, and therefore we're all vulnerable to a gaggle of influences that encourage us to exercise less-than-helpful eating behaviors that prioritize our right-now wants over our long-term goals. But when we understand the nature of our noshing tendencies and stumbling blocks, then we can figure out how to manage them. *That's the goal here*, and it's a moving target. The good news is you now have what you need—the tools, the strategies, and some recipes—to be able to navigate through these challenges gracefully, even when they shift.

The most reliable way to create the future you want is to first envision it and then work at it, a little bit at a time, every single day. Ultimately, the endgame is not about achieving perfection or always choosing your long-term aim over your short-term desire. Instead, it's to make food decisions that reflect what you really want for yourself while knowing how and when to loosen the reins so you can stay healthy, happy, and balanced for the long haul. *That's* the fairy tale—and you've *so* got this!

Acknowledgments

They say you shouldn't meet folks you admire, because it's often a tragic letdown. I respectfully disagree. GP, I am eternally grateful for your continued support and this opportunity with Goop Press. Thank you for cracking the door open for me, as you've done for so many women.

There are countless others to thank for their support for this book. In particular, I'd like to shout out the following individuals.

To J.L. Stermer, my literary agent, a fierce advocate, clip art lover and all-around delicious human, I couldn't imagine a better person in my corner. Thank you for all that you do, and for caring so deeply about me and this project.

A big thank you to Stacey Colino, my coach on this project, for your invaluable guidance throughout the writing process. I'm grateful to my meticulous editor, Katherine Stopa, for your passion and care. To the whole Grand Central team for the opportunity of a lifetime and for making the whole process so enjoyable. To Sarah Pelz, who helped shape this project in its early stages. To Hal Hershfield, whom I deeply admire, for graciously allowing me to feature his future self-continuity scale. And to Andie Yamagami, for your beautiful recipe.

Thank you to Elise Loehnen, an unbelievable badass, for being a believer in this book from the very start and for helping make it happen. My thanks to Kiki Koroshetz, an exceptionally gifted and thoughtful editor, book lover, and friend. To Jasmine, Alex, Thea, and Kate and the whole GOOP editorial and marketing team, thank you.

To my husband, Andrew, who is without a doubt my biggest champion and confidant in life.

To my pals, who read drafts, bounced ideas, and cheered me on from the beginning, in particular Alaina and Matthew, Eliza, Tasi, Nick A., Holly, Crystal, Mark D., Raina, Tanya E., Laurel, Erica, Puck, Marde, Leslie S., Amy B., Jenni K., Claire C., Carol and Andrew, Tara and Tucker, Dana and Mark F., Stacey and Henry, and Meaghan and Grant. To Danielle, for all your hard work helping me test these recipes, and for teaching me what it means to be a boss. To Julie, for everything. To my clients, who've trusted me with their obstacles, without whom there'd be no book.

To my parents for the unconditional love, anatomy coloring books, and also for sending me to cooking camp. Thanks to the Moores and Becky Moore, my second mom growing up, and an incredible cook. To two stand-up gentlemen from my formative years: Mr. Cunningham, my 7th grade science teacher, and Wayne Rickert, my high school rowing coach. To Judy and Isabelle, and of course Enrique, who I so wish I could share this with.

But honestly, thank *you*; I am seriously humbled to live on your shelves (digital and otherwise).

Select Bibliography

Introduction

Inzlicht, Michael, and Jennifer N. Gutsell. "Running on empty: Neural signals for self-control failure." *Psychological Science* 18, no. 11 (2007): 933–37. doi: https://doi.org/10.1111/j.1467-9280.2007.02004.x.

Stanley, Elizabeth A. "Neuroplasticity, mind fitness, and military effectiveness." *Bio-Inspired Innovation and National Security*. Ed. Robert E. Armstrong, Mark D. Drapeau, Cheryl A. Loeb, and James L. Valdes. Washington DC: National Defense University Press, 2010: 257–79. doi: http://www18.georgetown.edu/data/people/es63/publication-35451.pdf.

Chapter 1: Time to Have *The Talk* with Yourself

Adam, Tanja C., and Elissa S. Epel. "Stress, eating and the reward system." *Physiology & Behavior* 91, no. 4 (2007): 449–58. doi: https://doi.org/10.1016/j.physbeh.2007.04.011.

Adams, Claire E., and Mark R. Leary. "Promoting self–compassionate attitudes toward eating among restrictive and guilty eaters." *Journal of Social and Clinical Psychology* 26, no. 10 (2007): 1120–44. doi: http://psycnet.apa.org/doi/10.1521/jscp.2007.26.10.1120.

Bennett, Michael, and Sarah Bennett. *F*ck Feelings: One Shrink's Practical Advice for Managing All Life's Impossible Problems*. New York: Simon & Schuster, 2015.

Bublitz, Melissa G. *Why did I eat that? Perspectives on food decision making and dietary restraint*. The University of Wisconsin-Milwaukee, 2011. doi: http://dx.doi.org/10.1016%2Fj.jcps.2010.06.008.

Cruwys, Tegan, Kirsten E. Bevelander, and Roel C.J. Hermans. "Social modeling of eating: A review of when and why social influence affects food intake and choice." *Appetite* 86 (2015): 3–18. doi: https://doi.org/10.1016/j.appet.2014.08.035.

Exline, Julie J., Anne L. Zell, Ellen Bratslavsky, Michelle Hamilton, and Anne Swenson. "People-pleasing through eating: Sociotropy predicts greater eating in response to perceived social pressure." *Journal of Social and Clinical Psychology* 31, no. 2 (2012): 169–93. doi: http://guilfordjournals.com/doi/abs/10.1521/jscp.2012.31.2.169.

Fedoroff, Ingrid C., Janet Polivy, and C. Peter Herman. "The effect of pre-exposure to food cues on the eating behavior of restrained and unrestrained eaters." *Appetite* 28, no. 1 (1997): 33–47. doi: https://doi.org/10.1006/appe.1996.0057.

McGonigal, Kelly. *The Willpower Instinct: How Self-Control Works, Why It Matters, and What You Can Do to Get More of It.* New York: Avery, 2012.

Rubin, Gretchen. *Better Than Before: What I Learned About Making and Breaking Habits—to Sleep More, Quit Sugar, Procrastinate Less, and Generally Build a Happier Life.* New York: Crown Publishers, 2015.

Tice, Dianne M., Ellen Bratslavsky, and Roy F. Baumeister. "Emotional distress regulation takes precedence over impulse control: If you feel bad, do it!" *Journal of Personality and Social Psychology* 80, no. 1 (2001): 53–65. doi: http://dx.doi.org/10.1037/0022-3514.80.1.53.

van den Bos, Ruud, and Denise de Ridder. "Evolved to satisfy our immediate needs: Self-control and the rewarding properties of food." *Appetite* 47, no. 1 (2006): 24–29. doi: https://doi.org/10.1016/j.appet.2006.02.008.

Westenhoefer, Joachim, Petra Broeckmann, Anne-Kathrin Münch, and Volker Pudel. "Cognitive control of eating behavior and the disinhibition effect." *Appetite* 23, no. 1 (1994): 27–41. doi: http://psycnet.apa.org/doi/10.1006/appe.1994.1032.

Chapter 2: Cutting to the Core of Your Emotional Hang-ups Around Food

Adams, Claire E., and Mark R. Leary. "Promoting self-compassionate attitudes toward eating among restrictive and guilty eaters." *Journal of Social and Clinical Psychology* 26, no. 10 (2007): 1120–44. doi: http://psycnet.apa.org/doi/10.1521/jscp.2007.26.10.1120.

Baumeister, Roy F., and John Tierney. *Willpower: Rediscovering the Greatest Human Strength.* New York: Penguin Books, 2011.

Bove, Caron F., and Jeffery Sobal. "Body weight relationships in early marriage: Weight relevance, weight comparisons, and weight talk." *Appetite* 57, no. 3 (2011): 729–42. doi: https://dx.doi.org/10.1016%2Fj .appet.2011.08.007.

Bublitz, Melissa G. *Why did I eat that? Perspectives on food decision making and dietary restraint.* The University of Wisconsin-Milwaukee, 2011. doi: http://dx.doi.org/10.1016%2Fj.jcps.2010.06.008.

Burnette, Jeni L., and Eli J. Finkel. "Buffering against weight gain following dieting setbacks: An implicit theory intervention." *Journal of Experimental Social Psychology* 48, no. 3 (2012): 721–25. doi: https:// doi.org/10.1016/j.jesp.2011.12.020.

Crum, Alia J., William R. Corbin, Kelly D. Brownell, and Peter Salovey. "Mind over milkshakes: Mindsets, not just nutrients, determine ghrelin response." *Health Psychology* 30, no. 4 (2011): 424–429. doi: https://doi.org/10.1037/a0023467.

Fox, Robin. Food and Eating: An Anthropological Perspective. Social Issues Research Centre. Oxford, UK. Available online at http:// www.sirc.org/publik/food_and_eating_0.html.

Lethbridge, Jessica, Hunna J. Watson, Sarah J. Egan, Helen Street, and Paula R. Nathan. "The role of perfectionism, dichotomous thinking, shape and weight overvaluation, and conditional goal setting in eating disorders." *Eating Behaviors* 12, no. 3 (2011): 200–206. doi: https://doi.org/10.1016/j.eatbeh.2011.04.003.

Louis, Meryl Reis, and Robert I. Sutton. "Switching cognitive gears: From habits of mind to active thinking." *Human Relations* 44, no. 1 (1991): 55–76. doi: http://psycnet.apa.org/doi/10.1177/001872679104400104.

Mann, Traci. *Secrets from the Eating Lab: The Science of Weight Loss, the Myth of Willpower, and Why You Should Never Diet Again.* New York: Harper Wave, 2015.

McFarlane, Traci, Janet Polivy, and C. Peter Herman. "Effects of false weight feedback on mood, self-evaluation, and food intake in restrained and unrestrained eaters." *Journal of Abnormal Psychology* 107, no. 2 (1998): 312–18. doi: http://dx.doi.org/10.1037/0021-843X.107.2.312.

McGinnis, J. Michael et al. "Factors Shaping Food and Beverage Consumption of Children and Youth," *Food Marketing to Children and Youth: Threat or Opportunity?* Washington, DC: National Academies Press, 2006.

McGonigal, Kelly. *The Willpower Instinct: How Self-Control Works, Why It Matters, and What You Can Do to Get More of It.* New York: Avery, 2012.

Polivy, Janet, and C. Peter Herman. "Dieting and binging: A causal analysis." *American Psychologist* 40, no. 2 (1985): 193–201. doi: http://dx.doi.org/10.1037/0003-066X.40.2.193.

Prinsen, Sosja, Catharine Evers, and Denise de Ridder. "Oops I did it again: Examining self-licensing effects in a subsequent self-regulation dilemma." *Applied Psychology: Health and Well-Being* 8, no. 1 (2016): 104–26. doi: https://doi.org/10.1111/aphw.12064.

Rubin, Gretchen. *Better Than Before: What I Learned About Making and Breaking Habits—to Sleep More, Quit Sugar, Procrastinate Less, and Generally Build a Happier Life.* New York: Crown Publishers, 2015.

Sirois, Fuschia M., Ryan Kintner, and Jameson K. Hirsch. "Self-compassion, affect, and health-promoting behaviors." *Health Psychology* 34, no. 6 (2015): 661. doi: https://doi.org/10.1037/hea0000158.

Thompson, D'Arcy. *On Growth and Form.* New York: Cambridge University Press, 1942. Available online at https://archive.org/details/ongrowthform00thom.

Wagner, Dylan D., and Todd F. Heatherton. "Self-regulation and its failure: The seven deadly threats to self-regulation." *APA Handbook of Personality and Social Psychology* 1 (2015): 805–42. doi: http://psycnet.apa.org/doi/10.1037/14341-026.

Chapter 3: Meet Your Future Self

Ariely, Dan. "Self control: Dan Ariely at TEDxDuke," TED Video, posted April 2011, https://www.youtube.com/watch?v=PPQhj6ktYSo.

Bartels, Daniel M., and Oleg Urminsky. "On intertemporal selfishness: How the perceived instability of identity underlies impatient consumption." *Journal of Consumer Research* 38.1 (2011): 182–98. doi: http://dx.doi.org/10.1086/658339.

Hershfield, Hal E. "Future self-continuity: How conceptions of the future self transform intertemporal choice." *Annals of the New York Academy of Sciences* 1235 (2011): 30. doi: https://dx.doi.org/10.1111/j.1749-6632.2011.06201.x.

Hershfield, Hal E., Daniel G. Goldstein, William F. Sharpe, Jesse Fox, Leo Yeykelis, Laura L. Carstensen, and Jeremy N. Bailenson. "Increasing saving behavior through age-progressed renderings of the future self." *Journal of Marketing Research* 48, no. SPL (2011): S23–S37. doi: https://dx.doi.org/10.1509/jmkr.48.SPL.S23.

Hershfield, Hal E., G. Elliott Wimmer, and Brian Knutson. "Saving for the future self: Neural measures of future self-continuity predict temporal discounting." *Social Cognitive and Affective Neuroscience* 4, no. 1 (2009): 85–92. doi: https://doi.org/10.1093/scan/nsn042.

Hershfield, Hal E., Tess Garton, Kacey Ballard, Gregory R. Samanez-Larkin, and Brian Knutson. "Don't stop thinking about tomorrow: Individual differences in future self-continuity account for saving." *Judgment and Decision Making* 4, no. 4 (2009): 280–86. doi: http://halhershfield.com/wp-content/uploads/2016/06/Ersner-Hershfield_Garton_Ballard_Samanez-Larkin_Knutson_2009_JDM.pdf.

McGonigal, Kelly. *The Willpower Instinct: How Self-Control Works, Why It Matters, and What You Can Do to Get More of It.* New York: Avery, 2012.

O'Donoghue, Ted, and Matthew Rabin. "Doing it now or later." *American Economic Review* (1999): 103–24. doi: http://www.jstor.org/stable/116981.

Rubin, Gretchen. *Better Than Before: What I Learned About Making and Breaking Habits—to Sleep More, Quit Sugar, Procrastinate Less, and Generally Build a Happier Life.* New York: Crown Publishers, 2015.

van Gelder, Jean-Louis, Hal E. Hershfield, and Loran F. Nordgren. "Vividness of the future self predicts delinquency." *Psychological Science* 24, no. 6 (2013): 974–80. doi: https://dx.doi.org/10.1177/0956797612465197.

Chapter 4: Tune In to Your True Desires

Abramson, Edward. *Body Intelligence: Lose Weight, Keep It Off, and Feel Great About Your Body Without Dieting.* New York: McGraw-Hill, 2005.

Arnsten, Amy F.T. "Stress signalling pathways that impair prefrontal cortex structure and function." *Nature Reviews Neuroscience* 10, no. 6 (2009): 410–22. doi: https://dx.doi.org/10.1038/nrn2648.

Greeson, Jeffrey M. "Mindfulness research update: 2008." *Complementary Health Practice Review* 14, no. 1 (2009): 10–18. doi: https://dx.doi.org/10.1177%2F1533210108329862.

Heatherton, Todd F. "Neuroscience of self and self-regulation." *Annual Review of Psychology* 62 (2011): 363–90. doi: https://dx.doi.org/10.1146%2Fannurev.psych.121208.131616.

Higgs, Suzanne, and Jessica E. Donohoe. "Focusing on food during lunch enhances lunch memory and decreases later snack intake." *Appetite* 57, no. 1 (2011): 202–6. doi: https://dx.doi.org/10.1016/j.appet.2011.04.016.

Higgs, Suzanne, and Morgan Woodward. "Television watching during lunch increases afternoon snack intake of young women." *Appetite* 52, no. 1 (2009): 39–43. doi: https://doi.org/10.1016/j.appet.2008.07.007.

Holmes, Hannah. *Quirk: Brain Science Makes Sense of Your Particular Personality.* New York: Random House, 2011.

Inzlicht, Michael, Elliot Berkman, and Nathaniel Elkins-Brown. "The neuroscience of 'ego depletion'." *Social Neuroscience: Biological Approaches to Social Psychology* (2016): 101–23. doi: https://www.researchgate.net/profile/Elliot_Berkman/publication/273805571_The_neuroscience_of_ego_depletion_or_How_the_brain_can_help_us_understand_why_self-_control_seems_limited/links/550ddb6f0cf2128741675f8e.pdf.

Mann, Traci, and Andrew Ward. "To eat or not to eat: Implications of the attentional myopia model for restrained eaters." *Journal of Abnormal Psychology* 113, no. 1 (2004): 90–98. doi: https://dx.doi.org/10.1037/0021-843X.113.1.90.

Oldham-Cooper, Rose E., Charlotte A. Hardman, Charlotte E. Nicoll, Peter J. Rogers, and Jeffrey M. Brunstrom. "Playing a computer game during lunch affects fullness, memory for lunch, and later snack intake." *The American Journal of Clinical Nutrition* 93, no. 2 (2011): 308–13. doi: https://doi.org/10.3945/ajcn.110.004580.

Polivy, Janet, C. Peter Herman, Rick Hackett, and Irka Kuleshnyk. "The effects of self-attention and public attention on eating in restrained and unrestrained subjects." *Journal of Personality and Social Psychology* 50, no. 6 (1986): 1253–60. doi: http://psycnet.apa .org/doi/10.1037/0022-3514.50.6.1253.

Stanley, Elizabeth A. "Neuroplasticity, mind fitness, and military effectiveness." *Bio-Inspired Innovation and National Security.* Ed. Robert E. Armstrong, Mark D. Drapeau, Cheryl A. Loeb, and James L. Valdes. Washington DC: National Defense University Press, 2010: 257–79. doi: http://www18.georgetown.edu/data/people/ es63/publication-35451.pdf.

Tribole, Evelyn and Elyse Resch. *Intuitive Eating: A Revolutionary Program That Works*, 3rd ed. New York: St. Martin's Griffin, 2012.

Wansink, Brian, Koert Van Ittersum, and James E. Painter. "Ice cream illusions: Bowls, spoons, and self-served portion sizes." *American Journal of Preventive Medicine* 31, no. 3 (2006): 240–43. doi: https:// doi.org/10.1016/j.amepre.2006.04.003.

Chapter 5: Take the Pressure Off

Baumeister, Roy F., Ellen Bratslavsky, Mark Muraven, and Dianne M. Tice. "Ego depletion: Is the active self a limited resource?" *Journal of Personality and Social Psychology* 74, no. 5 (1998): 1252–65. doi: http://psycnet.apa.org/index.cfm?fa=buy .optionToBuy&id=1998-01923-011.

Baumeister, Roy F., and John Tierney. *Willpower: Rediscovering the Greatest Human Strength.* New York: Penguin Books, 2011.

Crockett, Molly J., Barbara R. Braams, Luke Clark, Philippe N. Tobler, Trevor W. Robbins, and Tobias Kalenscher. "Restricting temptations: Neural mechanisms of precommitment." *Neuron* 79, no. 2 (2013): 391–401. doi: https://dx.doi.org/10.1016/j.neuron.2013.05.028.

Goldsmith, Marshall. *Triggers: Creating Behavior That Lasts—Becoming the Person You Want to Be.* New York: Crown Business, 2015.

Kurth-Nelson, Zeb, and A. David Redish. "Don't let me do that!—Models of precommitment." *Frontiers in Neuroscience* 6 (2012): 138. doi: https://dx.doi.org/10.3389/fnins.2012.00138.

Levitin, Daniel J. *The Organized Mind: Thinking Straight in the Age of Information Overload.* New York: Plume, 2014.

Stites, Shana D., S. Brook Singletary, Adeena Menasha, Clarissa Cooblall, Donald Hantula, Saul Axelrod, Vincent M. Figueredo, and Etienne J. Phipps. "Pre-ordering lunch at work: Results of the what-to-eat-for lunch study." *Appetite* 84 (2015): 88–97. doi: https://doi.org/10.1016/j.appet.2014.10.005.

Vartanian, Lenny R., Kristin M. Kernan, and Brian Wansink. "Clutter, chaos, and overconsumption: The role of mind-set in stressful and chaotic food environments." *Environment and Behavior* 49, 2 (2016): 215–23. doi: http://dx.doi.org/10.1177%2F0013916516628178.

Vohs, Kathleen D., Roy F. Baumeister, Brandon J. Schmeichel, Jean M. Twenge, Noelle M. Nelson, and Dianne M. Tice. "Making choices impairs subsequent self-control: A limited-resource account of decision making, self-regulation, and active initiative." *Journal of Personality and Social Psychology* 94, no. 5 (2008): 883–98. doi: https://dx.doi.org/10.1037/0022-3514.94.5.883.

Wood, Wendy, and David T. Neal. "A new look at habits and the habit-goal interface." *Psychological Review* 114, no. 4 (2007): 843–63. doi: https://doi.org/10.1037/0033-295X.114.4.843.

Chapter 6: Get Your Hormones Working for You with the Food Therapist Plan

Christianson, Alan. *The Adrenal Reset Diet: Strategically Cycle Carbs and Proteins to Lose Weight*, Balance Hormones, and Move from Stressed to Thriving. New York: Harmony, 2014.

Cordain, Loren. The Paleo Diet: *Lose Weight and Get Healthy by Eating the Foods You Were Designed to Eat* (revised ed.). Boston: Houghton Mifflin Harcourt, 2011.

Dallman, Mary F., Norman C. Pecoraro, and Susanne E. la Fleur. "Chronic stress and comfort foods: Self-medication and abdominal obesity." *Brain, Behavior, and Immunity* 19, no. 4 (2005): 275–80. doi: https://doi.org/10.1016/j.bbi.2004.11.004.

Feinman, Richard D., and Eugene J. Fine. "'A calorie is a calorie' violates the second law of thermodynamics." *Nutrition Journal* 3, no. 1 (2004): 9. doi: https://dx.doi.org/10.1186%2F1475-2891-3-9.

Gottfried, Sara. *The Hormone Reset Diet: Heal Your Metabolism to Lose Up to 15 Pounds in 21 Days.* New York: HarperOne, 2015.

Hu, T., L. Yao, K. Reynolds, T. Niu, S. Li, P. K. Whelton, J. He, and L. Bazzano. "The effects of a low-carbohydrate diet on appetite: A randomized controlled trial." *Nutrition, Metabolism and Cardiovascular Diseases* 26, no. 6 (2016): 476–88. doi: https://doi.org/10.1016/j.numecd.2015.11.011.

Hyman, Mark. *Eat Fat, Get Thin: Why the Fat We Eat Is the Key to Sustained Weight Loss and Vibrant Health.* New York: Little, Brown and Company, 2016.

Lam, Sze Kwan, and Tzi Bun Ng. "Lectins: Production and practical applications." *Applied Microbiology and Biotechnology* 89, no. 1 (2011): 45–55. doi: https://doi.org/10.1007/s00253-010-2892-9.

Ludwig, David. *Always Hungry? Conquer Cravings, Retrain Your Fat Cells, and Lose Weight Permanently.* New York: Grand Central Life & Style, 2016.

Masley, Steven, and Jonny Bowden. *Smart Fat: Eat More Fat. Lose More Weight. Get Healthy Now.* New York: HarperOne, 2016.

Nickols-Richardson, Sharon M., Mary Dean Coleman, Joanne J. Volpe, and Kathy W. Hosig. "Perceived hunger is lower and weight loss is greater in overweight premenopausal women consuming a low-carbohydrate/high-protein vs high-carbohydrate/low-fat diet." *Journal of the American Dietetic Association* 105, no. 9 (2005): 1433–37. doi: https://doi.org/10.1016/j.jada.2005.06.025.

Shamay-Tsoory, Simone G., Meytal Fischer, Jonathan Dvash, Hagai Harari, Nufar Perach-Bloom, and Yechiel Levkovitz. "Intranasal administration of oxytocin increases envy and schadenfreude (gloating)." *Biological Psychiatry* 66, no. 9 (2009): 864–70. doi: https://doi.org/10.1016/j.biopsych.2009.06.009.

Sharma, Alka, and Salil Sehgal. "Effect of processing and cooking on the antinutritional factors of faba bean (Vicia faba)." *Food Chemistry* 43, no. 5 (1992): 383–85. doi: https://doi.org/10.1016/0308 -8146(92)90311-O.

Teta, Jade, and Keoni Teta. *Lose Weight Here: The Metabolic Secret to Target Stubborn Fat and Fix Your Problem Areas.* New York: Rodale, 2015.

Turner, Natasha. *The Hormone Diet: A 3-Step Program to Help You Lose Weight, Gain Strength, and Live Younger Longer.* New York: Rodale, 2009.

Willett, Walter C., and Rudolph L. Leibel. "Dietary fat is not a major determinant of body fat." *The American Journal of Medicine* 113, no. 9 (2002): 47–59. doi: https://doi.org/10.1016/S0002-9343(01)00992-5.

Chapter 8: Keep the Magic Alive

Guinard, Jean-Xavier, and Rossella Mazzucchelli. "The sensory perception of texture and mouthfeel." *Trends in Food Science & Technology* 7, no. 7 (1996): 213–19. doi: https://doi.org/10.1016/0924 -2244(96)10025-X.

Habib, Reza. "On the relation between conceptual priming, neural priming, and novelty assessment." *Scandinavian Journal of Psychology* 42, no. 3 (2001): 187–95. doi: https://doi.org/10.1111/1467-9450.00230.

Hyde, Robert J., and Steven A. Witherly. "Dynamic contrast: A sensory contribution to palatability." *Appetite* 21, no. 1 (1993): 1–16. doi: https://doi.org/10.1006/appe.1993.1032.

Maccotta, Luigi, and Randy L. Buckner. "Evidence for neural effects of repetition that directly correlate with behavioral priming." *Journal of Cognitive Neuroscience* 16, no. 9 (2004): 1625–32. doi: https://doi .org/10.1162/0898929042568451.

Masic, Una, and Martin R. Yeomans. "Umami flavor enhances appetite but also increases satiety." *The American Journal of Clinical Nutrition* 100, no. 2 (2014): 532–38. doi: http://ajcn.nutrition.org/ content/100/2/532.

McQuaid, John. *Tasty: The Art and Science of What We Eat*. New York: Scribner, 2015.

Morin-Audebrand, Léri, Jos Mojet, Claire Chabanet, Sylvie Issanchou, and Per Møller. "The role of novelty detection in food memory." *Acta Psychologica* 139, no. 1 (2012): 233–38. doi: https://doi.org/10.1016/j .actpsy.2011.10.003.

Ranganath, Charan, and Gregor Rainer. "Neural mechanisms for detecting and remembering novel events." Nature Reviews Neuroscience 4, no. 3 (2003): 193–202. doi: https://doi.org/10.1038/ nrn1052.

Schacter, Daniel L., Gagan S. Wig, and W. Dale Stevens. "Reductions in cortical activity during priming." *Current Opinion in Neurobiology* 17, no. 2 (2007): 171–76. doi: https://doi.org/10.1016/j .conb.2007.02.001.

Segnit, Niki. *The Flavor Thesaurus: A Compendium of Pairings, Recipes and Ideas for the Creative Cook*. New York: Bloomsbury, 2010.

Chapter 9: Get the %&^# Out of Your Own Way

Burnette, Jeni L., and Eli J. Finkel. "Buffering against weight gain following dieting setbacks: An implicit theory intervention." *Journal of Experimental Social Psychology* 48, no. 3 (2012): 721–25. doi: https:// doi.org/10.1016/j.jesp.2011.12.020.

De Witt Huberts, Jessie C., Catharine Evers, and Denise T.D. de Ridder. "'Because I am worth it': A theoretical framework and empirical review of a justification-based account of self-regulation failure." *Personality and Social Psychology Review* 18, no. 2 (2014): 119–38. doi: https://doi.org/10.1177/1088868313507533.

Effron, Daniel A. "Beyond 'Being Good Frees Us to Be Bad': Moral Self-Licensing and the Fabrication of Moral Credentials" (April 14, 2015). Paul A. M. van Lange and Jan-Willem van Prooijen (Eds.), *Cheating, Corruption, and Concealment: Roots of Unethical Behavior*. Cambridge, UK: Cambridge University Press, 2016. doi: https:// ssrn.com/abstract=2594403.

Effron, Daniel A., Benoît Monin, and Dale T. Miller. "The unhealthy road not taken: Licensing indulgence by exaggerating counterfactual sins." *Journal of Experimental Social Psychology* 49, no. 3 (2013): 573–78. doi: https://doi.org/10.1016/j.jesp.2012.08.012.

Hargrave, John S. *Mind Hacking: How to Change Your Mind for Good in 21 Days.* New York: Gallery Books, 2016.

Heatherton, Todd F., and Dylan D. Wagner. "Cognitive neuroscience of self-regulation failure." *Trends in Cognitive Sciences* 15, no. 3 (2011): 132–39. doi: https://doi.org/10.1016/j.tics.2010.12.005.

Hershfield, Hal E., Daniel G. Goldstein, William F. Sharpe, Jesse Fox, Leo Yeykelis, Laura L. Carstensen, and Jeremy N. Bailenson. "Increasing saving behavior through age-progressed renderings of the future self." *Journal of Marketing Research* 48, no. SPL (2011): S23–S37. doi: https://dx.doi.org/10.1509/jmkr.48.SPL.S23.

Louis, Meryl Reis, and Robert I. Sutton. "Switching cognitive gears: From habits of mind to active thinking." *Human Relations* 44, no. 1 (1991): 55–76. doi: http://psycnet.apa.org/doi/10.1177/001872679104400104.

McGonigal, Kelly. *The Willpower Instinct: How Self-Control Works, Why It Matters, and What You Can Do to Get More of It.* New York: Avery, 2012.

Mullen, Elizabeth, and Benoît Monin. "Consistency versus licensing effects of past moral behavior." *Annual Review of Psychology* 67 (2016): 363–85. doi: https://doi.org/10.1146/annurev-psych-010213-115120.

Myers, Christopher G., Bradley R. Staats, and Francesca Gino. "'My bad!' How internal attribution and ambiguity of responsibility affect learning from failure." *Working Paper, Harvard Business School* (April 18, 2014): 1–51. doi: http://citeseerx.ist.psu.edu/viewdoc/download?doi=10.1.1.1020.1380&rep=rep1&type=pdf.

Prinsen, Sosja, Catharine Evers, and Denise de Ridder. "Oops I did it again: Examining self-licensing effects in a subsequent self-regulation dilemma." *Applied Psychology: Health and Well-Being* 8, no. 1 (2016): 104–26. doi: https://doi.org/10.1111/aphw.12064.

Rosenzweig, Emily. "With eyes wide open: How and why awareness of the psychological immune system is compatible with its efficacy."

Perspectives on Psychological Science 11, no. 2 (2016): 222–38. doi: https://doi.org/10.1177/1745691615621280.

Rubin, Gretchen. *Better Than Before: What I Learned About Making and Breaking Habits—to Sleep More, Quit Sugar, Procrastinate Less, and Generally Build a Happier Life*. New York: Crown Publishers, 2015.

Sirois, Fuschia M., Jennifer Monforton, and Melissa Simpson. "'If only I had done better': Perfectionism and the functionality of counterfactual thinking." *Personality and Social Psychology Bulletin* 36, no. 12 (2010): 1675–92. doi: https://doi.org/10.1177/0146167210387614.

Tice, Dianne M., Roy F. Baumeister, Dikla Shmueli, and Mark Muraven. "Restoring the self: Positive affect helps improve self-regulation following ego depletion." *Journal of Experimental Social Psychology* 43, no. 3 (2007): 379–84. doi: https://doi.org/10.1016/j.jesp.2006.05.007.

Webb, Thomas L., and Paschal Sheeran. "Can implementation intentions help to overcome ego-depletion?" *Journal of Experimental Social Psychology* 39, no. 3 (2003): 279–86. doi: https://doi.org/10.1016/S0022-1031(02)00527-9.

Index

About the Author

Shira Lenchewski, M.S., R.D., is a registered dietitian and a nationally recognized nutrition expert. She is the resident nutritionist at goop and has been featured in magazines such as *Glamour, Seventeen, O, The Oprah Magazine*, and *Bon Appétit*, and on sites like Refinery29, Lenny Letter, Man Repeller, Well+GOOD, and POPSUGAR Fitness, among others. After completing her master's degree in clinical nutrition at New York University and her dietetic residency at the Mount Sinai Medical Center in New York City, Shira started her private practice. But she ditched the white lab coat to focus on helping clients untangle their complex relationships with food, so they can make conscious eating choices that serve their get-healthy goals while still enjoying delicious food in the process. She lives (and cooks a bunch) in Los Angeles, with her husband, Andrew. Visit her at shirard.com.